RENAL DIET RECIPES BOOK

Avoid Dialysis and

Manage All CKD Stages!

350+ Recipes All Low Sodium, Potassium, Phosphorus, and Sugar!

Beginners Guide Included!

By

Susan Cooper

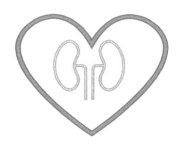

Renal Diet Cookbook

TABLE OF CONTENTS

INTRODUCTION 3

CHAPTER 1. THE RENAL DIET 4

CHAPTER 2. UNDERSTANDING KIDNEY DISEASE 6

CHAPTER 3. FOODS TO EAT AND TO AVOID...10

CHAPTER 4. FAQ: FREQUENTLY ASKED QUESTIONS 15

CHAPTER 5. BREAKFAST RECIPES..16

CHAPTER 6. LUNCH RECIPES..32

CHAPTER 7. DINNER RECIPES 52

CHAPTER 8. FISH AND SEAFOOD 69

CHAPTER 9. VEGETABLE RECIPES..81

CHAPTER 10. POULTRY RECIPES 92

CHAPTER 11. SOUP RECIPES..106

CHAPTER 12. EGGS AND DAIRY 116

CHAPTER 13. SALAD RECIPES 121

CHAPTER 14. DRINKS AND JUICES 126

CHAPTER 15. SMOOTHIES 130

CHAPTER 16. DESSERT RECIPES 135

28-DAY MEAL PLAN 156

CONCLUSION 158

INTRODUCTION

Human health hangs in the complete balance when all of its interconnected bodily mechanisms function properly in perfect sync. Without its significant organs functioning normally, the body soon suffers indelible damage. Kidney malfunction is one such example, and it is not only the entire water balance that is disturbed by kidney disease, but several other diseases also emerge due to this problem. Kidney disease is progressive, which means that it can eventually lead to permanent kidney damage if left unchecked and uncontrolled. This is why it is essential to control and manage the disease and stop its progress, which can be done through medicinal and natural means. While medication can only guarantee a thirty percent cure, a change in lifestyle and diet can prove miraculous with seventy percent guaranteed results. A kidney-friendly diet and lifestyle save the kidneys from mineral overload and help the medicines to work actively. Treatment without a good diet, therefore, proves futile. This kidney diet cookbook should highlight the basic facts about kidney diseases, symptoms, causes, and diagnosis.

This preliminary introduction can help readers clearly understand the problem; then, we will discuss the role of a kidney diet and a kidney-friendly lifestyle in curbing the diseases. And more. The book also contains several delicious kidney diet recipes that will ensure delicious flavors and good health.

Despite their small size, the kidneys perform several functions vital to the healthy functioning of the body.

These include:

> ➢ Filtering excess fluids and waste from the blood
> ➢ Creating the enzyme known as renin, which regulates blood pressure,
> ➢ Ensuring bone marrow creates red blood cells,
> ➢ Control calcium and phosphorus levels through absorption and excretion.

Unfortunately, when kidney disease reaches a chronic stage, these functions begin to stop working. However, with the proper treatment and lifestyle, you can manage your symptoms and continue to live well. This is even more applicable in the early stages of the disease. 10% of all adults over the age of 20 will experience some form of kidney disease in their lifetime. There are various treatments for kidney disease, depending on the cause of the disease.

According to international statistics, kidney (or renal) disease affects about 14% of the adult population. In the United States, approximately 661,000 Americans suffer from kidney dysfunction. Of these patients, 468,000 proceed to dialysis treatment, and the rest have an active kidney transplant.

High amounts of diabetes and heart disease are also linked to kidney dysfunction, and sometimes one condition, for example, diabetes, can cause the other.

With such a significant number of high rates, perhaps the best treatment course is dialysis contravention, making people depend on clinical medications and crisis facilities at any given occasion several times every week. That way, if your kidney has just given some indication of breaking down, you can prevent dialysis through a dietary routine, something we'll talk about in this book.

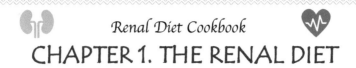
CHAPTER 1. THE RENAL DIET

THE BENEFITS OF RENAL DIET

If you have been diagnosed with kidney dysfunction, a proper diet is necessary to control toxic waste in the bloodstream. When toxic waste builds up in the system and increases fluid, chronic inflammation occurs, and we have a much higher chance of developing cardiovascular, bone, metabolic, or other health problems.

Since the kidneys cannot eliminate the waste on their own, which comes from food and drink, our system's only natural way is through this diet.

A kidney diet is beneficial during the early stages of kidney dysfunction and leads to the following benefits:

> ➢ Prevents excess fluid and waste build-up.
> ➢ Prevents the progression of renal dysfunction stages.
> ➢ Decreases the likelihood of developing other chronic health problems, e.g., heart disorders.
> ➢ It has a mild antioxidant function in the body, which keeps inflammation and inflammatory responses under control.

The above benefits are noticed once the patient follows the diet for at least a month and then continues it for more extended periods to avoid the stage where dialysis is needed. The severity of the diet depends on the current stage of the kidney disease; if, for example, one is in stage 3 or 4, one must follow a stricter diet and be careful about the foods that are allowed or prohibited.

NUTRIENTS YOU NEED

Potassium is a naturally occurring mineral found in almost all foods in varying amounts. Our bodies need a certain amount of potassium to help with muscle activity, electrolyte balance, and blood pressure regulation. However, if there is excess potassium in the system and the kidneys cannot excrete it (due to kidney disease), fluid retention and muscle spasms can occur.

Phosphorus is a trace mineral found in many foods, especially dairy products, meat, and eggs. It acts synergistically with calcium and vitamin D to promote bone health. However, when there is kidney damage, excess amounts of the mineral cannot be eliminated, causing bone weakness.

Sodium is what our bodies need to regulate fluid and electrolyte balance. It also plays a role in normal cell division in muscles and the nervous system. However, in kidney disease, sodium can quickly reach higher than normal levels, and the kidneys won't be able to excrete it, causing fluid buildup as a side effect. Those who also suffer from heart problems (as well) should limit their consumption because it may increase blood pressure.

Calories: when following a kidney diet, it is crucial to give yourself the correct number of calories: to fuel the system. The exact number of calories: to be consumed each day depends on your age, gender, general health, and kidney disease stage. However, in most cases, there are no strict limitations on calorie intake, as long as you get them from good sources that are low in sodium, potassium, and phosphorus. In general, doctors recommend a daily limit of between 1800-2100 calories: per day to keep your weight in the normal range.

Protein is an essential nutrient that our systems need to develop and generate new connective tissue, such as muscle, even during injury. Protein also helps stop bleeding and supports the immune system to fight infection. A healthy adult without kidney disease usually needs 40-65 grams of protein a day.

However, in a kidney diet, protein consumption is a complicated topic, as too much or too little can cause problems. When metabolized by our system, Protein also creates waste, which is usually processed by the kidneys. But when the kidneys are damaged or underperforming, these wastes remain in the system as in kidney disease. That's why patients in the more advanced CKD stages are advised to limit protein consumption as well.

Fats: Our systems need fats, particularly good fats, as a source of fuel and for other metabolic functions of the cells. A diet high in bad fats and trans or saturated fats can significantly increase your chances of developing heart problems, often with kidney disease. That's why most doctors advise their kidney patients to eat a diet that contains a decent amount of good fats and a low amount of trans (processed) or saturated fats.

Carbohydrates act as the primary and quick source of fuel for the body's cells. When we consume carbohydrates, our system converts them into glucose and then into energy to "fuel" our body's cells. Carbohydrates are generally not restricted in the kidney diet. However, some carbohydrates also contain dietary fiber, which helps regulate normal colon function and protect blood vessels from damage.

Dietary fiber is an essential element in our system that cannot be adequately digested, but it plays a key role in regulating our bowel movements and protecting blood cells. The fiber in the kidney diet is generally encouraged as it helps loosen stools, relieve constipation and bloating, and protect against damage to the colon. However, many patients do not get enough dietary fiber per day, as much of it is high in potassium or phosphorus. Fortunately, some good dietary fiber sources for CKD patients have lower amounts of these minerals than others.

Vitamins/Minerals: According to medical research, our systems need at least 13 vitamins and minerals to keep our cells fully active and healthy. However, patients with kidney disease are more likely to be depleted of water-soluble vitamins such as B-complex and vitamin C due to limited fluid intake. Therefore, supplementation of these vitamins and a renal diet program should help cover any vitamin deficiencies. Supplementation of fat-soluble vitamins such as vitamins A, K, and E can be avoided because they can build up quickly in the system and become toxic.

Fluids: when you are in an advanced kidney disease stage, fluids can build up quickly and lead to problems. While it's essential to keep your system well hydrated, you should avoid minerals like potassium and sodium, which can trigger further fluid buildup and cause a host of other symptoms.

NUTRIENT YOU NEED TO AVOID

Salt or sodium is known to be one of the most important ingredients that the kidney diet prohibits. This ingredient, though simple, can badly and strongly affect the body and especially the kidneys. Any excess of sodium cannot be filtered easily due to the weak condition of the kidneys. A massive accumulation of sodium can cause catastrophic results on your body. Potassium and phosphorus are also prohibited for kidney patients, depending on the stage of kidney disease.

CHAPTER 2. UNDERSTANDING KIDNEY DISEASE

Like all other parts of the body, human kidneys need a lot of care and attention to function effectively. It takes some simple and consistent measures to keep them healthy. Remember that no medicine can guarantee good health; only a better lifestyle can do that. Here are some of the practices that can keep your kidneys healthy for a lifetime.

1. Active lifestyle

An active routine is imperative for good health. This can include regular exercise, yoga or sports, and physical activities. The more you move your body, the more your metabolism improves. Water loss is compensated for by drinking more water, and this constantly drains all the toxins and waste from the kidneys. It also helps control blood pressure, cholesterol levels, and diabetes, which indirectly prevents kidney disease.

2. Control blood pressure

Consistently high blood pressure can cause glomerular damage. It is one of the leading causes, and every 3 out of 5 people who have hypertension also suffer from kidney problems. Normal human blood pressure is less than 120/80 mmHg. When there is a steady increase in this pressure to 140/100mmHg or more, it should be brought under control immediately. This can be done by minimizing salt intake, controlling cholesterol levels, and taking care of heart health. Before we delve further into the depths of the kidney diet, let's learn more about our kidneys and how they function. This basic understanding can ensure a better awareness of kidney disease. Our kidneys act as a filter; in fact, they are the body's natural filter, primarily filtering the blood that flows through them with high pressure. There is a kidney on both sides of the body; both work in sync to clean and purify the blood of the whole body on a regular and constant basis. The renal arteries entering the kidneys also pass through the membranes, which only let the harmful excretory products pass into the kidney's ureters and make the blood clean and purified. There is another vital function that the kidneys perform, which is to maintain the balance of water and electrolytes in the body. If our body has excess water, the kidneys release it through urination, and if our body is dehydrated, then more water is retained. This clever mechanism is only possible when a critical mineral balance is maintained within the kidney cells, as the release of water can only occur through osmosis.

Kidney function or renal function are the terms used to explain the functioning of the kidneys. A healthy individual is born with a pair of kidneys. Therefore, whenever one of the kidneys loses its function, it goes unnoticed due to the other kidney's function. But if the kidney function decreases further and reaches as low as 25 percent, it turns out to be serious for the patients. People who have only one functioning kidney need appropriate external therapy and, in the worst cases, a kidney transplant.

Kidney disease occurs when several kidney cells known as nephrons are partially or damaged and fail to filter blood that enters incorrectly. Gradual damage to kidney cells can occur due to various reasons; sometimes it is acid or toxic build-up within the kidney over time; sometimes, it is genetic or the result of other kidney-damaging diseases such as hypertension (high blood pressure) or diabetes.

3. Chronic Kidney Disease (CKD)

CKD or chronic kidney disease is the stage of kidney damage where they cannot properly filter blood. The term chronic is used to refer to gradual, long-term damage to an organ. Thus, chronic kidney disease develops after slow but progressive damage to the kidneys. Symptoms of this disease appear only when toxic waste begins to accumulate in the body. Therefore, such a stage should be prevented at all costs. Thus, early diagnosis of the disease proves to be significant. The sooner the patient realizes the situation's seriousness, the better measures he can take to curb the problem.

WHAT ARE THE CAUSES OF KIDNEY DISEASE?

There is never just one cause for the disease; several factors come into play and become the source of kidney deficiency. As mentioned before, these causes can include a person's genetics, certain other health disorders that can damage the kidneys, and the lifestyle a person lives. The following are the most commonly known causes of kidney disease:

* Heart disease
* Diabetes
* Hypertension (High blood pressure)
* Being around 60 years old
* Having kidney disease in the family
* Signs of renal disease

The good thing is that we can prevent the chronic phase of kidney disease by identifying the early signs of any form of kidney damage. Even when a person feels small changes in their body, they should consult an expert to confirm if it could lead to something serious. The following are some of the early signs of kidney damage:

- Tiredness or drowsiness
- Muscle cramps
- Loss of appetite
- Changes in the frequency of urination
- Swelling of hands and feet
- A feeling of itchiness
- Numbness
- The darkness of skin
- Trouble in sleeping
- Shortness of breath
- The feeling of nausea or vomiting

These symptoms can appear in combination with each other. They are general signs of body malfunction and should never be ignored. And if they are left unnoticed, they can lead to the worsening of the condition and can appear as:

- Back pain
- Abdominal pain
- Fever
- Rash
- Diarrhea
- Nosebleeds
- Vomiting

After seeing any of these symptoms, a person should immediately consult a health expert and prepare for the required lifestyle changes.

STAGES OF RENAL DISEASE

According to the National Kidney Foundation in the United States, kidney disease can be classified into five different progressive stages. These stages and their symptoms help the doctor devise appropriate therapy and guide the patient to take necessary routine life steps. The rate of kidney function says a lot about these stages. There is minimal loss of function in the early stages, increasing with each stage.

The eGFR is used as the standard criterion for measuring kidney function. eGFR stands for estimated Glomerular Filtration Rate. The rate at which waste material is transferred from the blood to the nephron tubes through the "glomerulus" - the kidney tissue's filtering membrane. The lower the glomerular filtration rate, the greater the kidney problem. A person's age, sex, race, and serum creatinine are entered into a mathematical formula to calculate his or her eGFR. The serum creatinine level is measured in a blood test. Creatinine is a waste product of the body that is produced by muscle activities. Healthy kidneys can remove all creatinine from the blood. A rising creatinine level is, therefore, a sign of kidney disease. If a person has an eGFR of less than 60 for three months, it means he or she is suffering from severe kidney problems. The five main stages of chronic kidney disease can be categorized as follows:

• Stage 1:

The first stage starts when the eGFR gets slightly higher than the standard value. In this stage, the eGFR can be equal to or greater than 90mL/min

• Stage 2:

The next stage arises when the eGFR starts to decline and ranges between 60 to 89 mL/min. It is best to control the progression of the disease at this point.

• Stage 3:

From this point on, the kidney disease becomes concerning for the patient as the eGFR drops to 30-59 mL/min. At this stage, consultation is essential for the health of the patient.

• Stage 4:

Stage 4 is also known as Severe Chronic Kidney Disease as the eGFR level drops to 15-29 mL/min.

• Stage 5:

The final and most critical phase of chronic renal disease is stage 5, where the estimated glomerular filtration rate gets as low as below 15 mL/min.

RENAL DISEASE DIAGNOSTIC TESTS

Besides identifying the symptoms of kidney disease, there are other better and more accurate ways to confirm the extent of loss of renal function. There are mainly two important diagnostic tests:

1. Urine test

The urine test indicates all kidney problems. Urine is the waste product of the kidney. When there is a loss of filtration or any kidney obstruction, the urine sample will indicate this through the number of excretory products present. Severe stages of chronic disease show some amount of protein and blood in the urine. Do not rely on self-tests; visit an authentic clinic for these tests.

2. Blood pressure and blood test

Another suitable way to check for kidney disease is to analyze the blood and its composition. A high amount of creatinine and other waste products in the blood indicates that the kidneys are not functioning properly. Blood pressure can also be indicative of kidney disease. When the water balance in the body is disturbed, it can cause high blood pressure. Hypertension can be both the cause and symptom of kidney disease and should be taken seriously.

HOW TO KEEP YOUR KIDNEYS HEALTHY

3. Hydration

Drinking more water and liquids without salt proves to be the life support for the kidneys. Water and fluids dilute the blood's consistency and lead to more urination; this, in turn, will get most of the excretions out of the body without much difficulty. Drinking at least eight glasses of water a day is essential. It is the lack of water that fatigues the kidneys and often hinders glomerular filtration. Water is the best option, but fresh juices without salt or preservatives are vital to kidney health. Keep them all in constant daily use.

4. Dietary changes

Certain foods are taken in excess that can cause kidney problems. In this regard, an extremely high protein diet, foods rich in sodium, potassium, and phosphorus can be harmful. People suffering from the early stages of kidney disease should reduce their intake, while those facing the critical stages of CKD should avoid them altogether. A well-planned renal diet can prove significant in this regard. It effectively limits all of these foods from the diet and promotes more fluids, water, organic fruits, and a low-protein meal plan.

5. No smoking/alcohol

Smoking and excessive alcohol use are other names for intoxication. Intoxication is another major cause of kidney disease or at least aggravates the condition. Smoking and drinking alcohol indirectly pollute the blood and body tissues, which leads to progressive kidney damage. Start gradually reducing alcohol consumption and smoking to a minimum.

6. Monitor the changes

Since the early signs of kidney disease are challenging to detect, it is essential to keep track of the changes occurring in your body. Even frequency of urination and loss of appetite are sufficient reasons to be cautious and concerned. Only a health expert can accurately diagnose the disease, but personal care and attention to small changes are of paramount importance to CKD.

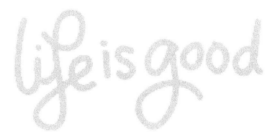

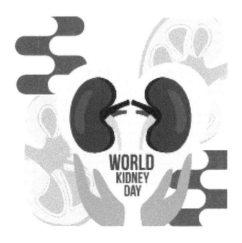

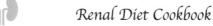
CHAPTER 3. FOODS TO EAT AND TO AVOID

FOOD TO EAT

The kidney diet aims to reduce the amount of waste in the blood. When people have kidney dysfunction, the kidneys are unable to properly remove and filter waste. When waste remains in the blood, it can affect the patient's electrolyte levels. With a renal diet, kidney function is promoted, and the progression of complete kidney failure is slowed.

The renal diet follows a low intake of protein, phosphorus, and sodium. It is necessary to consume high-quality protein and limit some fluids. For some people, limiting calcium and potassium is essential.

Promoting a renal diet, here are the substances that are critical to control:

SODIUM AND ITS ROLE IN THE BODY

Most natural foods contain sodium. Some people think that sodium and salt are interchangeable. However, salt is a compound of chloride and sodium. There can be both salt and sodium in other forms in the food we eat. Because of the added salt, processed foods include a higher level of sodium.

Along with potassium and chloride, sodium is one of the most important electrolytes in the body. The primary function of electrolytes is to control fluids as they leave and enter the body's cells and tissues.

With sodium:

* Blood volume and pressure are regulated.
* Muscle contraction and nerve function are regulated.
* The acid-base balance of the blood is regulated.
* The amount of fluid the body eliminates and keeps is balanced.

Why is it important to monitor sodium intake for people with kidney issues?

Since the kidneys of kidney disease patients are unable to reduce excess fluid and sodium from the body adequately, too much sodium might be harmful. As fluid and sodium build up in the bloodstream and tissues, they might cause:

* Edema: swelling in face, hands, and legs
* Increased thirst
* High blood pressure
* Shortness of breath
* Heart failure

The ways to monitor sodium intake:

➤ Avoid processed foods
➤ Be attentive to serving sizes.
➤ Read food labels
➤ Utilize fresh meats instead of processed
➤ Choose fresh fruits and veggies.
➤ Compare brands, choosing the ones with the lowest sodium levels.

- ➢ Utilize spices that do not include salt
- ➢ Ensure the sodium content is less than 400 mg per meal and not more than 150 mg per snack
- ➢ Cook at home, not adding salt
- ➢ Foods to eat with lower sodium content:
- ➢ Fresh meats, dairy products, frozen veggies, and fruits
- ➢ Fresh herbs and seasonings like rosemary, oregano, dill, lime, cilantro, onion, lemon, and garlic
- ➢ Corn tortilla chips, pretzels, no salt added crackers, unsalted popcorn

POTASSIUM AND ITS ROLE IN THE BODY

The main function of potassium is keeping muscles working correctly and the heartbeat regular. This mineral is responsible for maintaining electrolyte and fluid balance in the bloodstream. The kidneys regulate the proper amount of potassium in the body, expelling excess amounts in the urine.

Monitoring potassium intake:

- * Limit high potassium food
- * Select only fresh fruits and veggies
- * Limit dairy products and milk to 8 oz per day
- * Avoid potassium chloride
- * Read labels on packaged foods.
- * Avoid seasonings and salt substitutes with potassium.

Foods to eat with lower potassium:

- ➢ Fruits: watermelon, tangerines, pineapple, plums, peaches, pears, papayas, mangoes, lemons and limes, honeydew, grapefruit/grapefruit juice, grapes/grape juice, clementine/satsuma, cranberry juice, berries, and apples/ applesauce, apple juice
- ➢ Veggies: summer squash (cooked), okra, mushrooms (fresh), lettuce, kale, green beans, eggplant, cucumber, corn, onions (raw), celery, cauliflower, carrots, cabbage, broccoli (fresh), bamboo shoots (canned), and bell peppers
- ➢ Plain Turkish delights, marshmallows and jellies, boiled fruit sweets, and peppermints
- ➢ Shortbread, ginger nut biscuits, plain digestives
- ➢ Plain flapjacks and cereal bars
- ➢ Plain sponge cakes like Madeira cake, lemon sponge, jam sponge
- ➢ Corn-based and wheat crisps
- ➢ Whole grain crispbreads and crackers
- ➢ Protein and other foods (bread (not whole grain), pasta, noodles, rice, eggs, canned tuna, turkey (white meat), and chicken (white meat)

PHOSPHORUS AND ITS ROLE IN THE BODY

This mineral is essential in the development and maintenance of bones. Phosphorus helps in the development of organs and connective tissues and assists in the movement of muscles. Healthy kidneys can remove extra phosphorus. However, it is impossible with kidney dysfunction. High levels of phosphorus make bones weak by pulling calcium from the bones. It can lead to dangerous calcium deposits in the heart, eyes, lungs, and blood vessels.

Monitoring phosphorus intake:

* Pay attention to serving size
* Eat fresh fruits and veggies
* Eat smaller portions of foods that are rich in protein
* Avoid packaged foods
* Keep a food journal

Foods to eat with <u>low phosphorus</u> level:

* grapes, apples
* lettuce, leeks
* Carbs (white rice, corn, and rice Cereal, popcorn, pasta, crackers (not wheat), white bread)
* Meat (sausage, fresh meat)

PROTEIN

Damaged kidneys are unable to remove protein waste, so they accumulate in the blood. The amount of protein to consume differs depending on the stage of CKD. Protein is critical for tissue maintenance, and it is necessary to eat the proper amount of it according to the particular stage of kidney disease.

Sources of protein for vegetarians:

* Vegans (allowing only plant-based foods): Wheat protein and whole grains, nut butter, soy protein, yogurt or soy milk, cooked no salt added canned and dried beans and peas, unsalted nuts.
* Lacto vegetarians (allowing dairy products, milk, and plant-based foods): reduced-sodium or low-sodium cottage cheese.
* Lacto-Ovo vegetarians (allowing eggs, dairy products, milk, and plant-based foods): eggs.

FOOD TO AVOID

Food with <u>high sodium</u> content:

* Onion salt, marinades, garlic salt, teriyaki sauce, and table salt
* Pepperoni, bacon, ham, lunch meat, hot dogs, sausage, processed meats
* Ramen noodles, canned produce, and canned soups
* Marinara sauce, gravy, salad dressings, soy sauce, BBQ sauce, and ketchup
* Chex Mix, salted nuts, Cheetos, crackers, and potato chips
* Fast food

Food with a <u>high potassium</u> level:

* Fruits: dried fruit, oranges/orange juice, prunes/prune juice, kiwi, nectarines, dates, cantaloupe, bananas, black currants, damsons, cherries, grapes, and apricots.
* Vegetables: tomatoes/tomato sauce/tomato juice, sweet potatoes, beans, lentils, split peas, spinach (cooked), pumpkin, potatoes, mushrooms (cooked), chile peppers, chard, Brussels sprouts (cooked), broccoli (cooked), baked beans, avocado, butternut squash, and acorn squash.
* Protein and other foods: peanut butter, molasses, granola, chocolate, bran, sardines, fish, bacon, ham, nuts and seeds, yogurt, milkshakes, and milk.
* Coconut-based snacks, nut-based snacks, fudge, and toffee
* Cakes containing marzipan.

* Potato crisps.

Foods with <u>high phosphorus</u>:

* Dairy products: pudding, ice cream, yogurt, cottage cheese, cheese, and milk
* Nuts and seeds: sunflower seeds, pumpkin seeds, pecans, peanut butter, pistachios, cashews, and almonds
* Dried beans and peas: soybeans, split peas, refried beans, pinto beans, lentils, kidney beans, garbanzo beans, black beans, and baked beans.
* Meat: veal, turkey, liver, lamb, beef, bacon, fish, and seafood.
* Carbs: whole grain products, oatmeal, and bran cereals

RENAL DIET SHOPPING LIST

VEGETABLES:

* Arugula (raw)
* Alfalfa sprouts
* Bamboo shoots
* Asparagus
* Beans - pinto, wax, fava, green
* Bean sprouts
* Bitter melon (balsam pear)
* Beet greens (raw)
* Broccoli
* Broad beans (boiled, fresh)
* Cactus
* Cabbage - red, swamp, Napa/ Suey Choy, skunk
* Carrots
* Calabash
* Celery
* Cauliflower
* Chayote
* Celeriac (cooked)
* Collard greens
* Chicory
* Cucumber
* Corn
* Okra
* Onions

* Pepitas
* (Green) Peas
* Peppers
* Radish
* Radicchio
* Seaweed
* Rapini (raw)
* Shallots
* Spinach (raw)
* Snow peas
* Dandelion greens (raw)
* Daikon
* Plant Leaves
* Drumstick
* Endive
* Eggplant
* Fennel bulb
* Escarole
* Fiddlehead greens
* Ferns
* Hearts of Palm
* Irish moss
* Hominy
* Jicama, raw
* Leeks
* Kale(raw)
* Mushrooms (raw white)

* Lettuce (raw)
* Mustard greens
* Swiss chard (raw)
* Squash
* Turnip
* Tomatillos (raw)
* Watercress
* Turnip greens
* Wax beans
* Water chestnuts (canned)
* Winter melon
* Wax gourd
* Zucchini (raw)

FRUITS:

* Acerola Cherries
* Apple
* Blackberries
* Asian Pear
* Boysenberries
* Blueberries
* Cherries
* Casaba melon
* Clementine
* Chokeberries
* Crabapples
* Cloudberries

- Cranberries (fresh)
- Grapefruit
- Gooseberries
- Pomegranate
- Grapes
- Rambutan
- Quince
- Rhubarb
- Raspberries (fresh or frozen)
- Jujubes
- Golden Berry
- Kumquat
- Jackfruit
- Lingonberries
- Lemon

- Loganberries
- Lime
- Lychees
- Mango
- Mandarin orange
- Peach
- Pineapple
- Pear
- Plum
- Strawberries
- Rose-apple
- Tangerine
- Tangelo
- Watermelon

FRESH MEAT, SEAFOOD, AND POULTRY:
- Chicken
- Beef and Ground Beef
- Goat
- Duck
- Wild Game
- Pork
- Lamb
- Veal
- Turkey
- Fish

MILK, EGGS, AND DAIRY:

Milk:
- Milk (½-1 cup/day)

Non-Dairy Milk:
- Almond Fresh (Original, Unsweetened, Vanilla)
- Almond Breeze (Original, Vanilla, Vanilla Unsweetened, Original Unsweetened)
- Silk True Almond Beverage (Unsweetened Original, Original, Vanilla, Unsweetened Vanilla)
- Good Karma Flax Delight (Vanilla, Original, Unsweetened)
- Rice Dream Rice Drink (Vanilla Classic, Non-Enriched Original Classic)
- Silk Soy Beverage (Original, Vanilla, Unsweetened)
- Natura Organic Fortified Rice Beverage (Original, Vanilla)
- PC Organics Fortified Rice Beverage

Other Dairy Products:
- Non-Hydrogenated Margarine (Salt-Free or Regular)
- Butter (Unsalted or Regular)
- Whipping Cream
- Sour Cream
- Whipped Cream

CHAPTER 4. FAQ: FREQUENTLY ASKED QUESTIONS

Below are some of the most common questions about CKD.

What Are Precautions That I Can Take?

There are several steps you can take to protect your kidneys. Some include:
- ☞ Follow a kidney-friendly diet, such as the kidney diet
- ☞ Making sure to keep your blood pressure under control
- ☞ Quit smoking
- ☞ Keeping your blood glucose level under control

What Are Some Medications That I Should Avoid?

Some common medications to avoid that might lead to kidney diseases include:

- ✂ Over the counter painkillers
- ✂ Laxatives
- ✂ Enemas
- ✂ Anti-Inflammatory medicines
- ✂ Food supplements
- ✂ Vitamin and herbal medications

Always make sure to consult your Nephrologist before taking any over the counter medicine that might fall into any of the above categories.

Is There A Cure for CKD?

Unfortunately, no. Just like asthma, once you are affected by CKD, you can only keep it under control through proper management. There is no known permanent treatment at this time, but a proper diet can help you return to a lower CKD stage in some cases.

Is Cheese Allowed or Forbidden?

As a general rule, cheese should be avoided because it contains large amounts of phosphorus. However, some cheeses are less phosphorus-rich, such as goat cheese (the healthiest), cream cheese, Swiss cheese, natural cheese, etc. A pound or two of these once in a while won't hurt.

Are Soda Drinks Bad for a Kidney?

When considering sodas, be sure to especially avoid dark sodas, such as Pepsi or Coke, because they include phosphorus additives that are extremely harmful to your kidneys. Replace them with Cherry 7 Up, 7 Up, cream soda, ginger ale, sprite, etc. But even so, make sure you consume them in very small amounts, as little as possible. Avoiding these drinks would be best.

What Are Some Common Tests to Assess Kidney Functions?

Some common tests to check the condition of your kidney include:

- ☞ Blood tests that specifically look for BUN, Electrolytes, and Serum Creatinine.
- ☞ Urine tests that check for Glomerular Filtration rate and Microalbumin.
- ☞ Imaging tests such as renal ultrasound, CT Scan, or MRI.
- ☞ Kidney biopsy, where a small part of your kidney is removed by a needle to know if it is affected.

While some people with kidney disease need more potassium, others need less. Depending on how well your kidneys are functioning, your potassium need may vary.

CHAPTER 5. BREAKFAST RECIPES

1. BREAKFAST SALAD FROM GRAINS AND FRUITS

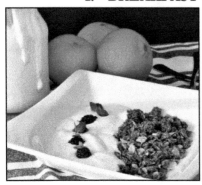

Preparation Time: 5 min.

Cooking Time: 15 min.

Servings: 6

Nutrition:

Calories: 187

Carbs: 47.3g

Protein: 10.9g

Fats: 2.4g

Potassium: 532mg

Sodium: 117mg

Ingredients:

- 1 8-oz low fat vanilla yogurt
- 1 cup raisins
- 1 orange
- 1 Red delicious apple
- 1 Granny Smith apple
- ¾ cup bulgur
- ¾ cup quick cooking brown rice
- ¼ tsp. salt
- 3 cups water

Directions:

1. On high fire, place a large pot and bring water to a boil.
2. Add bulgur and rice. Lower fire to a simmer and cooks for ten min. while covered.
3. Turn off fire, set aside for 2 min. while covered.
4. In baking sheet, transfer and evenly spread grains to cool.
5. Meanwhile, peel oranges and cut into sections. Chop and core apples.
6. Once grains are cool, transfer to a large serving bowl along with fruits.
7. Add yogurt and mix well to coat.
8. Serve and enjoy.

2. FRENCH TOAST WITH APPLESAUCE

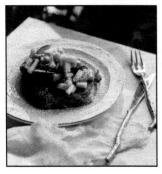

Preparation Time: 5 min.

Cooking Time: 15 min.

Servings: 6

Nutrition - Per Serving: Calories: 57

Carbs: 6g

Protein: 4g

Fats: 4g

Phosphorus: 69mg

Potassium: 88mg

Sodium: 43mg

Ingredients:

- ¼ cup unsweetened applesauce
- ½ cup milk
- 1 tsp. ground cinnamon
- 2 eggs
- 2 tbsp. white sugar
- 6 slices whole wheat bread

Directions:

1. Mix well applesauce, sugar, cinnamon, milk and eggs in a mixing bowl.
2. Dip the bread into applesauce mixture until wet, take note that you should do this one slice at a time.

3. On medium fire, heat a nonstick skillet greased with cooking spray.
4. Add soaked bread one at a time and cook for 2-3 min. per side or until lightly browned.
5. Serve and enjoy.

3. BAGELS FOR LOVERS

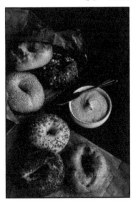

Preparation Time: 5 min.

Cooking Time: 25 min.

Servings: 8

Nutrition - Per Serving:

Calories: 221

Carbs: 42g

Protein: 7g

Fats: 3.1 g

Phosphorus: 130mg

Potassium: 166mg

Sodium: 47mg

Ingredients:
- 2 tsp. yeast
- 1 ½ tbsp. olive oil
- 1 ¼ cups bread flour
- 2 cups whole wheat flour
- 1 tbsp. vinegar
- 2 tbsp. honey
- 1 ½ cups warm water

Directions:
1. In a bread machine, mix all ingredients, and then process on dough cycle.
2. Once done or end of cycle, create 8 pieces shaped like a flattened ball.
3. Using your thumb, you must create a hole at the center of each then create a donut shape.
4. In a greased baking sheet, place donut-shaped dough then covers and let it rise about ½ h.
5. Prepare about 2 inches of water to boil in a large pan.
6. In a boiling water, drop one at a time the bagels and boil for 1 min., then turn them once.
7. Remove them and return them to baking sheet and bake at 350°F (175°C) for about 20 to 25 min. until golden brown.

4. CORNBREAD WITH SOUTHERN TWIST

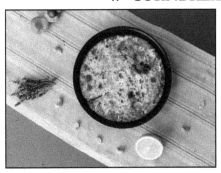

Preparation Time: 15 min.

Cooking Time: 60 min.

Servings: 8

Nutrition - Per Serving: Calories: 166

Carbs: 35g

Protein: 5g

Fats: 1g

Phosphorus: 79mg

Potassium: 122mg

Sodium: 34mg

Ingredients:
- 2 tbsp. shortening
- 1 ¼ cups skim milk
- ¼ cup egg substitute
- 4 tbsp. sodium free baking powder

☞ ½ cup flour   ☞ 1 ½ cups cornmeal

Directions:

1. Prepare 8 x 8-inch baking dish or a black iron skillet then add shortening.
2. Put the baking dish or skillet inside the oven on 425oF, once the shortening has melted that means the pan is hot already.
3. In a bowl, add milk and egg then mix well.
4. Take out the skillet and add the melted shortening into the batter and stir well.
5. Pour mixture into skillet after mixing all ingredients.
6. Cook the cornbread for 15-20 min. until it is golden brown.

5. GRANDMA'S PANCAKE SPECIAL

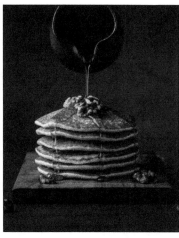

Preparation Time: 5 min.

Cooking Time: 15 min.

Servings: 3

Nutrition - Per Serving:

Calories: 167

Carbs: 50g

Protein: 11g

Fats: 11g

Phosphorus: 176mg

Potassium: 215mg

Sodium: 70mg

Ingredients:

☞ 1 tbsp. oil
☞ 1 cup milk
☞ 1 egg
☞ 2 tsp. sodium free baking powder
☞ 2 tbsp. sugar
☞ 1 ¼ cups flour

Directions:

6. Mix all the dry ingredients such as the flour, sugar and baking powder.
7. Combine oil, milk and egg in another bowl. Once done, add them all to the flour mixture.
8. Make sure that as your stir the mixture, blend them until slightly lumpy.
9. In a hot greased griddle, pour-in at least ¼ cup of the batter to make each pancake.
10. To cook, ensure that the bottom is a bit brown, then turn and cook the other side, as well.

7. VERY BERRY SMOOTHIE

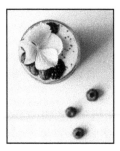

Preparation Time: 3 min.

Cooking Time: 5 min.

Servings: 2

Nutrition - Per Serving:

Calories: 464

Carbs: 111g

Protein: 8g; Fats: 4g

Phosphorus: 132mg

Potassium: 843mg

Sodium: 16mg

Ingredients:

- 2 quarts water
- 2 cups pomegranate seeds
- 1 cup blackberries
- 1 cup blueberries

Directions:

1. Mix all ingredients in a blender.
2. Puree until smooth and creamy.
3. Transfer to a serving glass and enjoy.

8. PASTA WITH INDIAN LENTILS

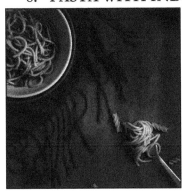

Preparation Time: 5 min.

Cooking Time: 0 min.

Servings: 6

Nutrition - Per Serving: Calories: 175

Carbs: 40g

Protein: 3g; Fats: 2g

Phosphorus: 139mg

Potassium: 513mg

Sodium: 61mg

Ingredients:

- ¼-½ cup fresh cilantro (chopped)
- 3 cups water
- 2 small dry red peppers (whole)
- 1 tsp. turmeric
- 1 tsp. ground cumin
- 2-3 cloves garlic (minced)
- 1 can diced tomatoes (w/juice)
- 1 large onion (chopped)
- ½ cup dry lentils (rinsed)
- ½ cup orzo or tiny pasta

Directions:

1. Combine all ingredients in the skillet except for the cilantro then boil on medium-high heat.
2. Ensure to cover and slightly reduce heat to medium-low and simmer until pasta is tender for about 35 min.
3. Afterwards, take out the chili peppers then add cilantro and top it with low-fat sour cream.

9. APPLE PUMPKIN MUFFINS

Preparation Time: 15 min.   **Cooking Time:** 20 min.   **Servings**: 12

Ingredients:

- 1 cup all-purpose flour
- 1 cup wheat bran
- 2 tsp. Phosphorus Powder
- 1 cup pumpkin purée
- ¼ cup honey
- ¼ cup olive oil
- 1 egg
- 1 tsp. vanilla extract
- ½ cup cored diced apple

Directions:

1. Preheat the oven to 400°F.
2. Line 12 muffin cups with paper liners.
3. Stir together the flour, wheat bran, and baking powder, mix this in a medium bowl.
4. In a small bowl, whisk together the pumpkin, honey, olive oil, egg, and vanilla.
5. Stir the pumpkin mixture into the flour mixture until just combined.
6. Stir in the diced apple.
7. Spoon the batter in the muffin cups.

8. Bake for about 20 min., or until a toothpick inserted in the center of a muffin comes out clean.

Nutrition - Per Serving: (1 muffin): Calories: 125; Total Fat: 5g; Saturated Fat: 1g; Cholesterol: 18mg; Sodium: 8mg; Carbs: 20g; Fiber: 3g; Phosphorus: 120mg; Potassium: 177mg; Protein: 2g

10. SPICED FRENCH TOAST

Preparation Time: 15 min.   **Cooking Time:** 12 min.   **Servings**: 4

Ingredients:

- 4 eggs
- ½ cup Homemade Rice Milk (here, or use unsweetened store-bought) or almond milk
- ¼ cup freshly squeezed orange juice
- 1 tsp. ground cinnamon
- ½ tsp. ground ginger
- Pinch ground cloves
- 1 tbsp. unsalted butter, divided
- 8 slices white bread

Directions:

1. Whisk eggs, rice milk, orange juice, cinnamon, ginger, and cloves until well blended in a large bowl. Melt half the butter in a large skillet. It should be in medium-high heat only.
2. Dredge four of the bread slices in the egg mixture until well soaked and place them in the skillet.
3. Cook the toast until golden brown on both sides, turning once, about 6 min. total.
4. Repeat with the remaining butter and bread.
5. Serve 2 pieces of hot French toast to each person.

Nutrition - Per Serving: Calories: 236; Total fat: 11g; Saturated fat: 4g; Cholesterol: 220mg; Sodium: 84mg; Carbs: 27g; Fiber: 1g; Phosphorus: 119mg; Potassium: 158mg; Protein: 11g

11. BREAKFAST TACOS

Preparation Time: 10 min.   **Cooking Time:** 10 min.   **Servings**: 4

Ingredients:

- 1 tsp. olive oil
- ½ sweet onion, chopped
- ½ red bell pepper, chopped
- ½ tsp. minced garlic
- 4 eggs, beaten
- ½ tsp. ground cumin
- Pinch red pepper flakes
- 4 tortillas
- ¼ cup tomato salsa

Directions:

1. Heat the oil in a large skillet in a medium heat only. Add the onion, bell pepper, and garlic, and sauté until softened, about 5 min.
2. Add the eggs, cumin, and red pepper flakes, and scramble the eggs with the vegetables until cooked through fluffy.
3. Spoon one-fourth of the egg mixture into each tortilla center, and top each with 1 tbsp. of salsa.
4. Serve immediately.

Nutrition - Per Serving: Calories: 211; Total fat: 7g; Saturated fat: 2g; Cholesterol: 211mg; Sodium: 346mg; Carbs: 17g; Fiber: 1g; Phosphorus: 120mg; Potassium: 141mg; Protein: 9g

12. RASPBERRY OVERNIGHT PORRIDGE

Preparation Time: Overnight   **Cooking Time:** 0 min.   **Servings**: 12

Ingredients:

Renal Diet Cookbook

- 1/3 cup of rolled oats
- ½ cup almond milk
- 1 tbsp. of honey
- 5-6 raspberries, fresh or canned and unsweetened

- 1/3 cup of rolled oats
- ½ cup almond milk
- 1 tbsp. of honey
- 5-6 raspberries, fresh or canned and unsweetened

Directions:

1. Combine the oats, almond milk, and honey in a mason jar and place into the fridge for overnight.
2. Serve the next morning with the raspberries on top.

Nutrition - Per Serving: Calories: 143.6 Carbs: 34.62 g Protein: 3.44 g Sodium: 77.88 mg Potassium: 153.25 mg Phosphorus: 99.3 mg Dietary Fiber: 7.56 g Fat: 3.91 g

13. CHEESY SCRAMBLED EGGS WITH FRESH HERBS

Preparation Time: 15 min. **Cooking Time:** 10 min. **Servings**: 4

Ingredients:

- 3 Eggs
- 2 Egg whites
- ½ cup Cream cheese
- ¼ cup Unsweetened rice milk

- 1 tbsp. green part only, Chopped scallion
- 1 tbsp., Chopped fresh tarragon
- 2 tbsp., Unsalted butter

- Ground black pepper to taste

Directions:

1. In a container, mix the eggs, egg whites, cream cheese, rice milk, scallions, and tarragon until mixed and smooth. Melt the butter in a skillet.

2. Pour in the egg mix and cook, stirring, for 5 min. or until the eggs are thick and curds creamy. Season with pepper and serve.

Nutrition - Per Serving: Calories: 221 Fat: 19g Carb: 3g Phosphorus: 119mg Potassium140mg Sodium193mg Protein8g

14. TURKEY AND SPINACH SCRAMBLE ON MELBA TOAST

Preparation Time: 2 min. **Cooking Time:** 15 min. **Servings**: 2

Ingredients:

- 1 tsp., Extra virgin olive oil
- 1 cup Raw spinach
- ½ clove, minced Garlic

- 1 tsp., grated Nutmeg
- 1 cup Cooked and diced turkey breast
- 4 slices, Melba toast

- 1 tsp., Balsamic vinegar

Directions:

1. Heat a pot over a source of heat and add oil.
2. Add turkey and heat through for 6 to 8 min. Add spinach, garlic, and nutmeg and stir-fry for 6 min. more.

3. Plate up the Melba toast and top with spinach and turkey scramble.
4. Drizzle with balsamic vinegar and serve.

Nutrition - Per Serving: Calories: 301 Fat: 19g Carb: 12g Phosphorus: 215mg Potassium: 269mg Sodium: 360mg Protein: 19g

15. VEGETABLE OMELET

Preparation Time: 15 min. **Cooking Time:** 10 min. **Servings**: 3

Ingredients:

- 4 Egg whites

- 1 Egg

- 2 tbsp., Chopped fresh parsley
- 2 tbsp., Water
- Olive oil spray
- ½ cup, Chopped and boiled red bell pepper
- ¼ cup, both green and white parts Chopped scallion
- Ground black pepper

Directions:

1. Whisk together the egg, egg whites, parsley, and water until well blended. Set aside.
2. Spray a skillet with olive oil spray and place over medium heat. Sauté the peppers and scallion for 3 min. or until softened.
3. Over the vegetables, you can now pour the egg and cook, swirling the skillet, for 2 min. or until the edges start to set. Cook until set.
4. Season with black pepper and serve.

Nutrition - Per Serving: Calories: 77 Fat: 3g Carb: 2g Phosphorus: 67mg Potassium: 194mg Sodium: 229mg Protein: 12g

16. MEXICAN STYLE BURRITOS

Preparation Time: 5 min. **Cooking Time:** 15 min. **Servings**: 2

Ingredients:

- 1 tbsp., Olive oil
- 2 Corn tortillas
- ¼ cup, chopped Red onion
- ¼ cup, chopped Red bell peppers
- ½, deseeded and chopped Red chili
- 2 Eggs
- 1 lime Juice
- 1 tbsp. chopped Cilantro

Directions:

1. Turn the broiler to medium heat and place the tortillas underneath for 1 to 2 min. on each side or until lightly toasted. Remove and keep the broiler on. Sauté onion, chili and bell peppers for 5 to 6 min. or until soft.
2. Place the eggs on top of the onions and peppers and place skillet under the broiler for 5-6 min. or until the eggs are cooked.
3. Serve half the eggs and vegetables on top of each tortilla and sprinkle with cilantro and lime juice to serve.

Nutrition - Per Serving: Calories: 202 Fat: 13g Carb: 19g Phosphorus: 184mg Potassium: 233mg Sodium: 77mg Protein: 9g

17. SWEET PANCAKES

Preparation Time: 10 min. **Cooking Time:** 5 min. **Servings**: 5

Ingredients:

- 1 cup, All-purpose flour
- 1 tbsp., Granulated sugar
- 2 tsp., Baking powder
- 2 Egg whites
- 1 cup, Almond milk
- 2 tbsp., Olive oil
- 1 tbsp., Maple extract

Directions:

1. Combine the flour, sugar and baking powder in a bowl. Make a well in the center and place to one side. Mx the egg whites, milk, oil, and maple extract, do this in another bowl.
2. Add the egg mixture to the well and gently mix until a batter is formed.

Heat skillet over medium heat.
3. Cook 2 min. on each side or until the pancake is golden only add 1/5 of the batter to the pan. Repeat with the remaining batter and serve.

Nutrition - Per Serving: Calories: 178 Fat Potassium: 126mg Fat: 5.6g Carb: 2.4g; Sodium: 297mg; Protein: 6g

18. BREAKFAST SMOOTHIE

Preparation Time: 15 min.   **Cooking Time:** 0 min.   **Servings**: 2

Ingredients:

- 1 cup Frozen blueberries
- ½ cup Pineapple chunks
- ½ cup English cucumber
- ½ Apple
- ½ cup Water

Directions:

1. Put the pineapple, blueberries, cucumber, apple, and water in a blender and blend until thick and smooth.
2. Pour into 2 glasses and serve.

Nutrition - Per Serving: Calories: 87 Fat: g Carb: 22g Phosphorus: 28mg Potassium: 192mg Sodium: 3mg Protein: 0.7g

19. BUCKWHEAT AND GRAPEFRUIT PORRIDGE

Preparation Time: 5 min.   **Cooking Time:** 20 min.   **Servings**: 2

Ingredients:

- ½ cup Buckwheat
- ¼, chopped Grapefruit
- 1 tbsp. Honey
- 1 ½ cups Almond milk
- 2 cups Water

Directions:

1. Boil water on the stove. Add the buckwheat and place the lid on the pan.
2. Simmer for 7 to 10 min., in a low heat. Check to ensure water does not dry out. Remove and set aside for 5 min., do this when most of the water is absorbed.
3. Drain excess water from the pan and stir in almond milk, heating through for 5 min. Add the honey and grapefruit. Serve.

Nutrition - Per Serving: Calories: 231 Fat: 4g Carb: 43g Phosphorus: 165mg Potassium: 370mg Sodium: 135mg

20. EGG AND VEGGIE MUFFINS

Preparation Time: 15 min.   **Cooking Time:** 20 min.   **Servings**: 4

Ingredients:

- Cooking spray
- 4 Eggs
- 2 tbsp. Unsweetened rice milk
- ½, chopped Sweet onion
- ½, chopped Red bell pepper
- Pinch red pepper flakes
- Pinch ground black pepper

Directions:

1. Preheat the oven to 350F. Spray 4 muffin pans with cooking spray. Set aside.
2. Whisk together the milk, eggs, onion, red pepper, parsley, red pepper flakes, and black pepper until mixed.
3. Pour the egg mixture into prepared muffin pans.
4. Bake until the muffins are puffed and golden, about 18 to 20 min. Serve

Nutrition - Per Serving: Calories: 84 Fat: 5g Carb: 3g Phosphorus: 110mg Potassium: 117mg Sodium: 75mg Protein:7g

21. BAKED CURRIED APPLE OATMEAL CUPS

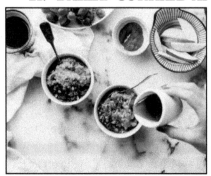

Preparation Time: 10 min.

Cooking Time: 20 min.

Servings: 6

Nutrition - Per Serving:

For 2 Oatmeal Cups:

Calories: 296;

Total fat: 10g

Saturated Fat: 1g

Sodium: 84mg

Phosphorus: 236mg

Potassium: 289mg

Carbs: 45g

Fiber: 6g

Protein: 8g,

Sugar: 11g

Ingredients:

- 3½ cups old-fashioned oats
- 3 tbsp. brown sugar
- 2 tsp. of your preferred curry powder
- 1/8 tsp. salt
- 1 cup unsweetened almond milk
- 1 cup unsweetened applesauce
- 1 tsp. vanilla
- ½ cup chopped walnuts

Directions:

1. Preheat the oven to 375°F. Then spray a 12-cup muffin tin with baking spray then set aside.
2. Combine the oats, brown sugar, curry powder, salt, and mix in a medium bowl.
3. Mix the milk, applesauce, and vanilla in a small bowl,
4. Stir the liquid ingredients into the dry ingredients and mix until just combined. Stir in the walnuts. Using a scant 1/3 cup for each divide the mixture among the muffin cups.
5. Bake this for 18 to 20 min. until the oatmeal is firm. Serve.

22. MOZZARELLA CHEESE OMELETTE

Preparation Time: 10 min.   **Cooking Time:** 5 min.   **Servings:** 1

Ingredients:

- 4 eggs, beaten
- 1/4 cup mozzarella cheese, shredded
- 4 tomato slices
- 1/4 tsp. Italian seasoning
- 1/4 tsp. dried oregano
- Pepper
- Salt

Directions:

1. In a small bowl, whisk eggs with salt.
2. Spray pan with cooking spray and heat over medium heat. Pour egg mixture into the pan and cook over medium heat. Once eggs are set then sprinkle oregano and Italian seasoning on top.
3. Arrange tomato slices on top of the omelet and sprinkle with shredded cheese.
4. Cook omelet for 1 min. Serve and enjoy.

Nutrition - Per Serving: Calories:285 Fat 19g Carbs 4g Sugar 3g Protein 25g Cholesterol 655mg; Sodium: 447 mg; Potassium: 386mg

23. SUN-DRIED TOMATO FRITTATA

Preparation Time: 10 min.   **Cooking Time:** 20 min.   **Servings:** 8

Ingredients:

- 12 eggs
- 1/2 tsp. dried basil
- 1/4 cup parmesan cheese, grated
- 2 cups baby spinach, shredded
- 1/4 cup sun-dried tomatoes, sliced
- Pepper
- Salt

Directions:

1. Preheat the oven to 425 F.
2. In a large bowl, whisk eggs with pepper and salt.
3. Add remaining ingredients and stir to combine.
4. Spray oven-safe pan with cooking spray.
5. Pour egg mixture into the pan and bake for 20 min.
6. Slice and serve.

Nutrition - Per Serving: Calories: 115 Fat 7 g Carbs 1 g Sugar 1 g Protein 10 g Cholesterol 250 mg; Sodium: 119 mg; Potassium: 144 mg

24. ITALIAN BREAKFAST FRITTATA

Preparation Time: 10 min.   **Cooking Time:** 45 min.   **Servings**: 4

Ingredients:

- 2 cups egg whites
- 1/2 cup mozzarella cheese, shredded
- 1 cup cottage cheese, crumbled
- 1/4 cup fresh basil, sliced
- 1/2 cup roasted red peppers, sliced
- Pepper
- Salt

Directions:

1. Preheat the oven to 375 F.
2. Add all ingredients into the large bowl and whisk well to combine.
3. Pour frittata mixture into the baking dish and bake for 45 min.
4. Slice and serve.

Nutrition - Per Serving: Calories: 131 Fat 2 g Carbs 5 g Sugar 2 g Protein 22 g Cholesterol 6 mg ; Sodium: 467 mg; Phosphorus: mg; Potassium: 295 mg

25. SAUSAGE CHEESE BAKE OMELETTE

Preparation Time: 10 min.   **Cooking Time:** 45 min.   **Servings**: 8

Ingredients:

- 10 eggs
- 2 cups cheddar cheese, shredded
- 1/2 cup salsa
- 1 lb ground sausage
- 1 1/2 cups coconut milk
- Pepper
- Salt

Directions:

1. Preheat the oven to 350 F.
2. Add sausage in a pan and cook until browned. Drain excess fat.
3. In a large bowl, whisk eggs and milk. Stir in cheese, cooked sausage, and salsa.
4. Pour omelet mixture into the baking dish and bake for 45 min.
5. Serve and enjoy.

Nutrition - Per Serving: Calories: 360 Saturated Fat: 24 g Carbs: 4 g Sugar: 2.6 g Protein: 28 g Cholesterol: 284 mg Sodium: 801 mg; Potassium: 436 mg

26. GREEK EGG SCRAMBLED

Preparation Time: 10 min.   **Cooking Time:** 10 min.   **Servings**: 2

Ingredients:

- 4 eggs
- 1/2 cup grape tomatoes, sliced
- 2 tbsp. green onions, sliced
- 1 bell pepper, diced
- 1 tbsp. olive oil
- 1/4 tsp. dried oregano
- 1/2 tbsp. capers
- 3 olives, sliced
- Pepper
- Salt

Directions:

1. Heat oil in a pan over medium heat.
2. Add green onions and bell pepper and cook until pepper is softened.
3. Add tomatoes, capers, and olives and cook for 1 min.
4. Add eggs and stir until eggs are cooked. Season with oregano, pepper, and salt.
5. Serve and enjoy.

Nutrition - Per Serving: Calories: 230 Fat: 17 g Carbs: 8 g Sugar: 5 g Protein: 12 g Cholesterol: 325 mg Sodium: 327mg; Potassium: 358mg

27. FETA MINT OMELETTE

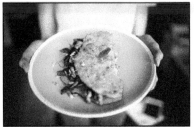

Preparation Time: 10 min.
Cooking Time: 5 min.
Servings: 2
Nutrition - Per Serving:

Calories: 275	Protein 20 g
Fat 20 g	Cholesterol 505 mg
Carbs 4 g	Sodium: 280mg
Sugar 2 g	Potassium: 187mg

Ingredients:

- 3 eggs
- 1/4 cup fresh mint, chopped
- 2 tbsp. coconut milk
- 1/2 tsp. olive oil
- 2 tbsp. feta cheese, crumbled
- Pepper
- Salt

Directions:

1. In a bowl, whisk eggs with feta cheese, mint, milk, pepper, and salt.
2. Heat olive oil in a pan over low heat.
3. Pour egg mixture in the pan and cook until eggs are set. Flip omelet and cook for 2 min. more. Serve and enjoy.

28. SAUSAGE CASSEROLE

Preparation Time: 10 min. **Cooking Time:** 50 min. **Servings**: 8

Ingredients:

- 12 eggs
- 1 lb. ground Italian sausage
- 2 1/2 tomatoes, sliced
- 3 tbsp. coconut flour
- 1/4 cup coconut milk
- 2 small zucchinis, shredded
- Pepper
- Salt

Directions:

1. Preheat the oven to 350 F.
2. Cook sausage in a pan until brown.
3. Transfer sausage to a mixing bowl.
4. Add coconut flour, milk, eggs, zucchini, pepper, and salt. Stir well.
5. Add eggs and whisk to combine.
6. Transfer bowl mixture into the casserole dish and top with tomato slices.
7. Bake for 50 min.
8. Serve and enjoy

Nutrition - Per Serving: Calories: 305 Fat: 21.8 g Carbs: 6.3 g Sugar: 3.3 g Protein: 19.6 g Cholesterol: 286 mg Sodium: 598mg; Potassium: 277mg

29. SIMPLE TURKEY BURRITOS FOR BREAKFAST

Preparation Time: 10 min. **Cooking Time:** 0 min. **Servings**: 8

Ingredients

- 1 lb. of ground turkey or 1 lb. of meatloaf of surplus turkey, diced in small cubes
- 8'6-inch burrito shells of flour
- 8 beaten and scrambled eggs
- ¼ cup canola oil
- ¼ cup diced bell peppers (yellow, green, or red)
- 2 tbsp. jalapeño peppers (seeded)
- ¼ cup diced onions
- 2 tbsp. chopped fresh scallions
- ½ tsp. chili powder
- 2 tbsp. chopped fresh cilantro
- ½ tsp. smoked paprika
- 1 cup shredded Cheddar cheese and Monterey Jack

Directions

1. Sauté the meatloaf, peppers, cilantro, onions, and scallions until translucent in half the liquid. Stir in the spices, then turn the heat off.
2. Set the pan over medium-high heat with another broad sauté pan and add the scrambled eggs and remaining oil.
3. Place equal quantities of meatloaf mix and vegetables, eggs, and cheese in the burrito shells, then roll and serve.

Nutrition - Per Serving: Calories 407 Protein 25 g Sodium 513 mg Phosphorus 359 mg Fiber 2 g Potassium 285 mg

30. BLUEBERRY MUFFINS

Preparation Time: 40 min.　　　**Cooking Time:** 30 min.　　　**Servings:** 12

Ingredients

- ½ cup butter (unsalted)
- 2 eggs
- 2 cups 1% milk
- 1 ¼ cups sugar
- 2 tsp. baking powder
- 2 cups flour
- ½ tsp. salt
- 2 tsp. sugar (for topping)
- 2 ½ cups blueberries

Directions

1. Mix the sugar and margarine until fluffy and creamy, utilizing a mixer at low speed.
2. One at a time, add the eggs and stir until mixed.
3. Sift the dry ingredients and add milk alternately. Mash and stir in 1/2 cup of blueberries by hand. Then add the leftover blueberries and mix them by hand.
4. Spray the top of the pan and muffin cups with vegetable oil. Put the muffins cups in a tin.
5. In each muffin cup, pile up the muffin mixture. Sprinkle the muffin tops with sugar.
6. Bake for 25–30 min. at 375° F. Before careful removal, cool in the pan for a maximum of 30 min.

Nutrition Per Serving: Calories 275 Protein 5 g Sodium 210 mg Phosphorus 100 mg Fiber 1.3g Potassium 121 mg

31. Stuffed Biscuits

Preparation Time: 30 min.　　　**Cooking Time:** 20 min.　　　**Servings:** 12

Ingredients

- 2 cups flour
- ½ tsp. baking soda
- 1 tbsp. sugar or honey
- 1 tbsp. lemon juice
- ¾ cup milk
- 8 tbsp. unsalted butter

Filling

- 1 cup shredded cheddar cheese
- 8 oz. or 1¼ chopped sodium bacon
- 4 eggs
- ¼ cup scallions (thinly sliced)

Directions

1. Preheat the oven to 425 ° F

Get the filling ready:

2. Slightly under-cooked scrambled eggs.
3. Get the bacon cooked until crispy.
4. Mix and set aside the four ingredients.

Get the dough prepared:

1. Combine all of the dried ingredients in a big bowl.

2. Slice with a fork or pastry knife the unsalted butter till pea-size or smaller. In the middle of the Mix, make a well and knead in the lemon juice and milk. Start preparing muffin tins with a lining or gently grease the bottom and sides with flour.
3. Scoop the muffin tins with 1/4 cup of Mix.
4. Bake for 10-12 min. or till golden brown at 425° F.

Nutrition Per Serving: Calories 330 Protein 11 g Sodium 329 mg Phosphorus 170 mg Fiber 1 g Potassium 152 mg

32. GREEN LETTUCE BACON BREAKFAST BAKE

Preparation Time: 10 min.   **Cooking Time:** 45 min.   **Servings:** 6

Ingredients:
- 10 eggs
- 3 cups baby green lettuce, chopped
- tbsp. olive oil
- 8 bacon slices, cooked and chopped
- Red bell peppers, sliced
- tbsp. chives, chopped
- Pepper
- Salt

Directions:
1. Preheat the oven to 350 F.
2. Spray a baking dish with cooking spray and set aside. Heat oil in a pan
3. Add green lettuce and cook until green lettuce wilted.
4. In a mixing bowl, whisk eggs and salt. Add green lettuce and chives and stir well.
5. Pour egg mixture into the baking dish.
6. Top with Red bell peppers and bacon and bake for 45 min. Serve and enjoy.

Nutrition – Per Serving: Calories 273 Fat 20.4g Carbs 3.1g Sugar 1.7g Protein 19.4g Cholesterol 301 mg

33. HEALTHY GREEN LETTUCE TOMATO MUFFINS

Preparation Time: 10 min. **Cooking Time**: 20 min. **Servings**: 12

Ingredients:
- 12 eggs
- 1/2 tsp. Italian seasoning
- 1 cup Red bell peppers, chopped
- 4 tbsp. water
- 1 cup fresh green lettuce, chopped
- Pepper
- Salt

Directions:
1. Preheat the oven to 350 F. Spray a muffin tray with cooking spray and set aside.
2. In a mixing bowl, whisk eggs with water, Italian seasoning, pepper, and salt.
3. Add green lettuce and Red bell peppers and stir well. Pour egg mixture into the prepared muffin tray and bake for 20 min.
4. Serve and enjoy.

Nutrition – Per Serving: Calories 67 Fat 4.5g Carbs 1g Sugar 0.8g Protein 5.7g Cholesterol 164 mg

34. CHICKEN EGG BREAKFAST MUFFINS

Preparation Time: 10 min.   **Cooking Time**: 15 min.   **Servings**: 12

Ingredients:
- 10 eggs
- 1 cup cooked chicken, chopped
- 3 tbsp. green onions, chopped
- 1/4 tsp. garlic powder
- Pepper
- Salt

Directions:
1. Preheat the oven to 400 F.
2. Spray a muffin tray with cooking spray and set aside. In a large bowl, whisk eggs with garlic powder, pepper, and salt.
3. Add remaining ingredients and stir well.
4. Pour egg mixture into the muffin tray and bake for 15 min.
5. Serve and enjoy.

Nutrition – Per Serving: Calories 71 Fat 4 g Carbs 0.4g Sugar 0.3g Protein 8g Cholesterol 145 mg

35. BREAKFAST EGG SALAD

Preparation Time: 10 min.   **Cooking Time**: 5 min.   **Servings**: 4

Ingredients:
- 6 eggs, hard-boiled, peeled and chopped
- 1 tbsp. fresh dill, chopped
- 4 tbsp. mayonnaise
- Pepper
- Salt

Directions:
1. Add all ingredients into the large bowl and stir to mix. Serve and enjoy.

Nutrition – Per Serving: Calories 140 Fat 10g Carbs 4g Sugar 1g Protein 8g Cholesterol 245 mg

36. VEGETABLE TOFU SCRAMBLE

Preparation Time: 10 min.   **Cooking Time**: 7 min.   **Servings**: 2

Ingredients:

- 1/2 block firm tofu, crumbled
- 1/4 tsp. ground cumin
- tbsp. turmeric
- cup green lettuce
- 1/4 cup zucchini, chopped
- tbsp. olive oil
- tomato, chopped
- tbsp. chives, chopped
- tbsp. coriander, chopped
- Pepper
- Salt

Directions:

2. Heat oil in a pan over medium heat
3. Add tomato, zucchini, and green lettuce and sauté for 2 min.
4. Add tofu, cumin, turmeric, pepper, and salt and sauté for 5 min. Top with chives, and coriander. Serve and enjoy.

Nutrition – Per Serving: Calories 101 Fat 8.5 g Carbs 5.1g Sugar 1.4g Protein 3.1g Cholesterol 0 mg

37. CHEESE COCONUT PANCAKES

Preparation Time: 10 min.   **Cooking Time**: 5 min.   **Servings**: 1

Ingredients:

- 2 eggs
- packet stevia
- 1/2 tsp. cinnamon
- oz. cream cheese
- tbsp. coconut flour
- 1/2 tsp. vanilla

Directions:

1. Add all ingredients into the bowl and blend until smooth.
2. Spray pan with cooking spray and heat over medium-high heat.
3. Pour batter on the hot pan and make two pancakes. Cook pancake until lightly brown from both the sides.
4. Serve and enjoy.

Nutrition – Per Serving: Calories 386 Fat 30g Carbs 12g Sugar 1g Protein 16g Cholesterol 389 mg

38. SCRAMBLED EGGS WITH FRESH HERBS

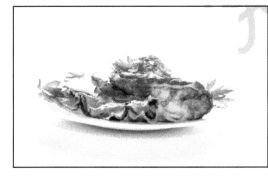

Preparation Time: 15 min.
Cooking Time: 10 min.
Servings: 4
Ingredients:

- Eggs – 3
- Egg whites – 2
- Cream cheese – 1/2 cup
- Unsweetened rice milk – 1/4 cup
- Chopped scallion – 1 Tbsp. green part only
- Chopped fresh tarragon – 1 Tbsp.
- Unsalted butter – 2 Tbsps.
- Ground black pepper to taste

Directions:

1. In a bowl, whisk the eggs, egg whites, cream cheese, rice milk, scallions, and tarragon until mixed and smooth.
2. Melt the butter in a skillet.
3. Pour in the egg mixture and cook, stirring, for 5 min. or until the eggs are thick and curds creamy.
4. Season with pepper and serve.

Nutrition – Per Serving: Calories: 221 Fat: 19g Carb: 3g Phosphorus: 119mg Potassium: 140mg Sodium: 193mg Protein: 8g

39. MIXED VEGETABLE BARLEY

Preparation time: 15 min.   **Cooking time**: 35 min.   **Servings**: 6

Ingredients:

- 1 tbsp. olive oil
- 1 medium sweet onion, chopped
- 2 tsp. minced garlic
- 2 cups fresh cauliflower florets
- 1 red bell pepper, diced
- 1 carrot, sliced
- ½ cup barley
- ½ cup white rice

- 2 cups water
- 1 tbsp. minced fresh parsley

Directions:

1. Heat the olive oil on a skillet over medium heat.
2. Sauté the garlic and onion up until softened, about 3 min. Stir in the cauliflower, bell pepper, and carrot, and sauté for 5 min.
3. Stir in the barley, rice, and water to a boil.
4. Cover, lower the heat and simmer until the liquid is absorbed and the barley and rice are tender, about 25 min. Serve topped with the parsley.

Nutrition: Calories: 156kcal Total fat: 3g Saturated fat: 0g Cholesterol: 0mg Sodium: 16mg Carbs: 30g Fiber: 4g Phosphorus: 83mg Potassium: 220mg Protein: 4g

40. SPICY SESAME TOFU

Preparation time: 15 min.　**Cooking time**: 10 min.　**Servings:** 6

Ingredients:

- 1 tbsp. toasted sesame oil
- 1 tbsp. grated peeled fresh ginger
- 2 tsp. minced garlic
- 2 red bell peppers, thinly sliced
- 1 (14-ounce) package tofu, drain and cut into cubes
- 2 cups quartered Bok choy
- 2 scallions, white and green parts, cut thinly on a bias
- 3 tbsp. low-sodium soy sauce
- 2 tbsp. freshly squeezed lime juice
- Pinch red pepper flakes
- 2 tbsp. chopped fresh cilantro
- 2 tbsp. toasted sesame seeds

Directions:

1. Heat the sesame oil in a skillet over medium heat. Add the ginger and garlic, and sauté until softened, about 3 min. Stir in the bell peppers and tofu, and gently sauté for about 3 min.
2. Add the Bok choy and scallions, and sauté until the Bok choy is wilted, about 3 min.
3. Add the soy sauce, lime juice, and red pepper flakes and toss to coat. Serve topped with cilantro and sesame seeds.

Nutrition: Calories: 80kcal Total fat: 3g Saturated fat: 0g Cholesterol: 0mg Sodium: 503mg Carbs: 4g Fiber: 1g Phosphorus: 88mg Potassium: 165mg Protein: 6g

41. MUSHROOM RICE NOODLES

Preparation time: 15 min.　**Cooking time**: 15 min.　**Servings**: 4

Ingredients:

- 4 cups rice noodles
- 2 tsp. toasted sesame oil
- 2 cups sliced wild mushrooms
- 2 tsp. minced garlic
- 1 red bell pepper, sliced
- 1 yellow bell pepper, sliced
- 1 carrot, julienned
- 2 scallions, white and green parts, sliced
- 1 tbsp. low-sodium soy sauce

Directions:

1. Prepare the rice noodles as said on the package instructions and set them aside.
2. Heat the sesame oil in a skillet over medium heat.
3. Sauté the red bell pepper, yellow bell pepper, carrot, and scallions until tender, about 5 min.
4. Stir together the soy sauce, and the noodles toss to coat. Serve.

Nutrition: Calories: 163kcal Total fat: 2g Saturated fat: 0g Cholesterol: 0mg Sodium: 199mg Carbs: 33g Fiber: 2g Phosphorus: 69mg Potassium: 200mg Protein: 2g

42. EGG FRIED RICE

Preparation time: 10 min.　**Cooking time**: 20 min.　**Servings**: 6

Ingredients:

- 1 tbsp. olive oil
- 1 tbsp. grated peeled fresh ginger
- 1 tsp. minced garlic
- 1 cup chopped carrots
- 1 scallion, white and green parts, chopped
- 2 tbsp. chopped fresh cilantro
- 4 cups cooked rice
- 1 tbsp. low-sodium soy sauce
- 4 eggs, beaten

Directions:

1. Heat the olive oil in a skillet over medium heat.
2. Add the ginger and garlic, and sauté until softened, about 3 min.
3. Add the carrots, scallion, and cilantro, and sauté until tender, about 5 min.
4. Stir in the soy sauce and rice, and sauté until the rice is well cooked for about 5 min.
5. Move the rice to the other side of the skillet and pour the eggs into space. Scramble the eggs and mix them with rice. Serve hot.

Nutrition: Calories: 204kcal Total fat: 6g Saturated fat: 1g Cholesterol: 141mg Sodium: 223mg Carbs: 29g Fiber: 1g Phosphorus: 120mg Potassium: 147mg Protein: 8g

43. VEGETABLE RICE CASSEROLE

Preparation time: 10 min. **Cooking time**: 50 min. **Servings**: 4

Ingredients:
- 1 tsp. olive oil
- ½ small sweet onion, chopped
- ½ tsp. minced garlic
- ½ cup chopped red bell pepper
- ¼ cup grated carrot
- 1 cup white basmati rice
- 2 cups of water
- ¼ cup grated Parmesan cheese
- Freshly ground black pepper

Directions:
1. Pre-heat the oven to 350°F
2. Heat the olive oil in a skillet over medium-high heat. Sauté onion and garlic until softened for about 3 min. Transfer the vegetables to a 9-by-9-inch baking dish and stir in the rice and water.
3. Cover the dish and bake until the liquid is absorbed 35 to 40 min.
4. Sprinkle the cheese on top and bake an additional 5 min to melt. Season the casserole with pepper and serve.

Nutrition: Calories: 224kcal Total fat: 3g Saturated fat: 1g Cholesterol: 6mg Sodium: 105mg Carbs: 41g Fiber: 2g Phosphorus: 118mg Potassium: 176mg Protein: 6g

44. FRENCH TOAST SPECIAL

Preparation time: 5 min. **Cooking time**: 8 min. **Servings**: 4

Ingredients:
- 4 slices white bread, cut in half diagonally
- 3 whole eggs and 1 egg white
- 1 cup plain almond milk
- 2 tbsp. canola oil
- 1 tsp. cinnamon

Directions:
1. Pre-heat your oven to 400°F/180°C. With the almond milk, beat the eggs.
2. Heat the oil in a pan.
3. Dip each bread slice/triangle into the egg and almond milk mixture.
4. Fry in a pan until golden brown.
5. Place the toasts in a baking dish and let cook in the oven for another 5 min.
6. Serve warm and drizzle with some honey, icing sugar, or cinnamon on top.

Nutrition: Calories: 293.75kcal Carbs: 25.3g Protein: 9.27g Sodium: 211g Potassium: 97mg Phosphorus: 165mg, Dietary Fiber: 12.3g Fat: 16.50g

CHAPTER 6. LUNCH RECIPES

45. SAUCY GARLIC GREENS

Preparation Time: 5 min.   **Cooking Time:** 20 min.   **Servings**: 4

Ingredients:

- 1 bunch of leafy greens
- Sauce
- ½ cup cashews soaked in water for 10 min.
- ¼ cup water
- 1 tbsp. lemon juice
- 1 tsp. coconut aminos
- 1 clove peeled whole clove
- 1/8 tsp. of flavored vinegar

Directions:

1. Make the sauce by draining and discarding the soaking water from your cashews and add the cashews to a blender.
2. Add fresh water, lemon juice, flavored vinegar, coconut aminos, garlic.
3. Blitz until you have a smooth cream and transfer to bowl.
4. Add ½ cup of water to the pot.
5. Place the steamer basket to the pot and add the greens in the basket.
6. Lock the lid and steam for 1 min.
7. Quick release the pressure.
8. Transfer the steamed greens to strainer and extract excess water.
9. Place the greens into a mixing bowl.
10. Add lemon garlic sauce and toss.

Nutrition - Per Serving: Calories: 77; Fat: 5g; Carbs: 0g; Protein: 2g; Phosphorus: 126mg; Potassium: 255mg; Sodium: 281mg

46. GARDEN SALAD

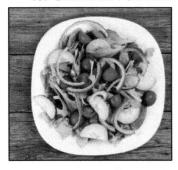

Preparation Time: 5 min.

Cooking Time: 20 min.

Servings: 6

Nutrition - Per Serving: Calories: 140

Fat: 4g	Phosphorus: 216mg
Carbs: 24g	Potassium: 185mg
Protein: 5g	Sodium: 141mg

Ingredients:

- 1-pound raw peanuts in shell
- 1 bay leaf
- 2 medium-sized chopped up tomatoes
- ½ cup diced up green pepper
- ½ cup diced up sweet onion
- ¼ cup finely diced hot pepper
- ¼ cup diced up celery
- 2 tbsp. olive oil
- ¾ tsp. flavored vinegar
- ¼ tsp. freshly ground black pepper

Directions:

1. Boil your peanuts for 1 min. and rinse them. The skin will be soft, so discard the skin. Add 2 cups of water to the Instant Pot. Add bay leaf and peanuts.
2. Lock the lid and cook on HIGH pressure for 20 min. Drain the water.
3. Take a large bowl and add the peanuts, diced up vegetables. Whisk in olive oil, lemon juice, pepper in another bowl.
4. Pour the mixture over the salad and mix.

47. SPICY CABBAGE DISH

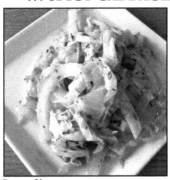

Preparation Time: 10 min.

Cooking Time: 4 hs

Servings: 4

Nutrition - Per Serving:

Calories: 197

Fat: 1g

Carbs: 14g

Protein: 3g

Phosphorus: 216mg

Potassium: 285mg

Sodium: 281mg

Ingredients:

- 2 yellow onions, chopped
- 10 cups red cabbage, shredded
- 1 cup plums, pitted and chopped
- 1 tsp. cinnamon powder
- 1 garlic clove, minced
- 1 tsp. cumin seeds
- ¼ tsp. cloves, ground
- 2 tbsp. red wine vinegar
- 1 tsp. coriander seeds
- ½ cup water

Directions:

1. Add cabbage, onion, plums, garlic, cumin, cinnamon, cloves, vinegar, coriander and water to your Slow Cooker. Stir well.
2. Place lid and cook on LOW for 4 hs.
3. Divide between serving platters.

48. EXTREME BALSAMIC CHICKEN

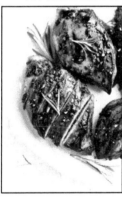

Preparation Time: 10 min.
Cooking Time: 35 min.
Servings: 4
Nutrition - Per Serving:

Calories: 546

Fat: 35g

Carbs: 11g

Protein: 44g

Phosphorus: 136mg

Potassium: 195mg

Sodium: 81mg

Ingredients:

- 3 boneless chicken breasts, skinless
- Sunflower seeds to taste
- ¼ cup almond flour
- 2/3 cups low-fat chicken broth
- 1 ½ tsp. arrowroot
- ½ cup low sugar raspberry preserve
- 1 ½ tbsp. balsamic vinegar

Directions:

1. Cut chicken breast into bite-sized pieces and season them with seeds.
2. Dredge the chicken pieces in flour and shake off any excess.
3. Take a non-stick skillet and place it over medium heat.
4. Add chicken to the skillet and cook for 15 min., making sure to turn them half-way through.
5.
6. Remove chicken and transfer to platter.
7. Add arrowroot, broth, raspberry preserve to the skillet and stir.
8. Stir in balsamic vinegar and reduce heat to low, stir-cook for a few min.
9. Transfer the chicken back to the sauce and cook for 15 min. more.
10. Serve and enjoy!

49. ENJOYABLE SPINACH AND BEAN MEDLEY

Preparation Time: 10 min. **Cooking Time:** 4 hs **Servings**: 4

Ingredients:

- 5 carrots, sliced
- 1 ½ cups great northern beans, dried
- 2 garlic cloves, minced
- 1 yellow onion, chopped
- Pepper to taste

- ½ tsp. oregano, dried
- 5 ounces baby spinach
- 4 ½ cups low sodium veggie stock
- 2 tsp. lemon peel, grated
- 3 tbsp. lemon juice

Directions:

1. Add beans, onion, carrots, garlic, oregano and stock to your Slow Cooker.
2. Stir well.
3. Place lid and cook on HIGH for 4 hs.

4. Add spinach, lemon juice and lemon peel.
5. Stir and let it sit for 5 min.
6. Divide between serving platters and enjoy!

Nutrition - Per Serving: Calories: 219; Fat: 8g; Carbs: 14g; Protein: 8g; Phosphorus: 216mg; Potassium: 285mg; Sodium: 131mg

50. TANTALIZING CAULIFLOWER AND DILL MASH

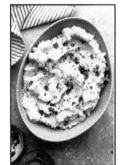

Preparation Time: 10 min.

Cooking Time: 6 hs

Servings: 6

Nutrition - Per Serving:

Calories: 207

Fat: 4g

Carbs: 14g

Protein: 3g

Phosphorus: 226mg

Potassium: 285mg

Sodium: 134mg

Ingredients:

- 1 cauliflower head, florets separated
- 1/3 cup dill, chopped
- 6 garlic cloves

- 2 tbsp. olive oil
- Pinch of black pepper

Directions:

1. Add cauliflower to Slow Cooker.
2. Add dill, garlic and water to cover them.
3. Place lid and cook on HIGH for 5 hs.
4. Drain the flowers.

5. Season with pepper and add oil, mash using potato masher.
6. Whisk and serve.

51. SECRET ASIAN GREEN BEANS

Preparation Time: 10 min. **Cooking Time:** 2 hs **Servings**: 10

Ingredients:

- 16 cups green beans, halved
- 3 tbsp. olive oil
- ¼ cup tomato sauce, salt-free

- ½ cup coconut sugar
- ¾ tsp. low sodium soy sauce
- Pinch of pepper

Directions:

1. Add green beans, coconut sugar, pepper tomato sauce, soy sauce, oil to your Slow Cooker.

2. Stir well.
3. Place lid and cook on LOW for 3 hs.
4. Divide between serving platters and serve.
5. Enjoy!

Nutrition - Per Serving: Calories: 200 Fat: 4g Carbs: 12g Protein: 3g Phosphorus: 216mg; Potassium: 285mg; Sodium: 131mg

52. EXCELLENT ACORN MIX

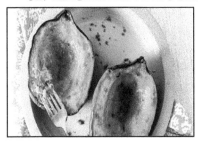

Preparation Time: 10 min.
Cooking Time: 7 hs
Servings: 10
Nutrition - Per Serving:

Calories: 200
Fat: 3g
Carbs: 15g
Protein: 2g

Phosphorus: 211mg
Potassium: 243m
Sodium: 203mg

Ingredients:

- 2 acorn squash, peeled and cut into wedges
- 16 ounces cranberry sauce, unsweetened
- ¼ tsp. cinnamon powder
- Pepper to taste

Directions:

1. Add acorn wedges to your Slow Cooker.
2. Add cranberry sauce, cinnamon, raisins and pepper.
3. Stir.
4. Place lid and cook on LOW for 7 hs.
5. Serve and enjoy!

53. CRUNCHY ALMOND CHOCOLATE BARS

Preparation Time: 10 min.   **Cooking Time:** 2 hs 30 min.   **Servings**: 12

Ingredients:

- 1 egg white
- ¼ cup coconut oil, melted
- 1 cup coconut sugar
- ½ tsp. vanilla extract
- 1 tsp. baking powder
- 1 ½ cups almond meal
- ½ cup dark chocolate chips

Directions:

1. Take a bowl and add sugar, oil, vanilla extract, egg white, almond flour, baking powder and mix it well.
2. Fold in chocolate chips and stir.
3. Line Slow Cooker with parchment paper.
4. Grease.
5. Add the cookie mix and press on bottom.
6. Place lid and cook on LOW for 2 hs 30 min.
7. Take cookie sheet out and let it cool.
8. Cut in bars and enjoy!

Nutrition - Per Serving: Calories: 200; Fat: 2g; Carbs: 13g; Protein: 6g; Phosphorus: 136mg; Potassium: 285mg; Sodium: 281mg

54. GOLDEN EGGPLANT FRIES

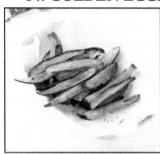

Preparation Time: 10 min.
Cooking Time: 15 min.
Servings: 8
Nutrition - Per Serving:

Calories: 212
Fat: 15.8g
Carbs: 12.1g
Protein: 8.6g

Phosphorus: 116mg
Potassium: 185mg
Sodium: 121mg

Ingredients:

- 2 eggs
- 2 cups almond flour
- 2 tbsp. coconut oil, spray
- 2 eggplant, peeled and cut thinly
- Sunflower seeds and pepper

Directions:

1. Preheat your oven to 400 F.
2. Take a bowl and mix with sunflower seeds and black pepper.
3. Take another bowl and beat eggs until frothy.
4. Dip the eggplant pieces into the eggs.
5. Then coat them with the flour mixture.
6. Add another layer of flour and egg.
7. Then, take a baking sheet and grease with coconut oil on top.
8. Bake for about 15 min.
9. Serve and enjoy!

55. LETTUCE AND CHICKEN PLATTER

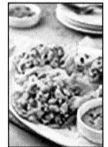

Preparation Time: 10 min.
Cooking Time: 0 min.
Servings: 6
Nutrition - Per Serving:

Calories: 296
Fat: 21g
Carbs: 9g

Protein: 18g
Phosphorus: 146mg
Potassium: 205mg

Sodium: 221mg

Ingredients:

- 2 cups chicken, cooked and coarsely chopped
- ½ head iceberg lettuce, sliced and chopped
- 1 celery rib, chopped
- 1 medium apple, cut
- ½ red bell pepper, deseeded and chopped
- 6-7 green olives, pitted and halved
- 1 red onion, chopped
- For dressing
- 1 tbsp. raw honey
- 2 tbsp. lemon juice
- Salt and pepper to taste

Directions:

1. Cut the vegetables and transfer them to your Salad Bowl. Add olives.
2. Chop the cooked chicken and transfer to your Salad bowl.
3. Prepare dressing by mixing the ingredients listed under Dressing.
4. Pour the dressing into the Salad bowl.
5. Toss and enjoy!

56. GREEK LEMON CHICKEN BOWL

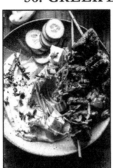

Preparation Time: 10 min.

Cooking Time: 15 min.

Servings: 6

Nutrition - Per Serving:

Calories: 520

Fat: 33g

Carbs: 31g

Protein: 30g

Phosphorus: 216m

Potassium: 285mg

Sodium: 281mg

Ingredients:

- 2 cups chicken, cooked and chopped
- 2 cans chicken broth, fat free
- 2 medium carrots, chopped
- ¼ tsp. pepper
- 2 tbsp. parsley, snipped
- ¼ cup lemon juice
- 1 can cream chicken soup, fat free, low sodium
- ½ cup onion, chopped
- 1 garlic clove, minced

Directions:

1. Take a pot and add all the ingredients except parsley into it.
2. Season with salt and pepper.
3. Bring the mix to a boil over medium-high heat.
4. Reduce the heat and simmer for 15 min.
5. Garnish with parsley.
6. Serve hot and enjoy!

57. SPICY CHILI CRACKERS

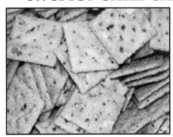

Preparation Time: 15 min.

Cooking Time: 60 min.

Servings: 10

Nutrition - Per Serving:

Carbs: 2.8g; Fiber: 1g; Protein: 1.6g; Fat: 4.1g

Phosphorus: 216mg; Potassium: 285mg; Sodium: 191mg

Ingredients:

- ¾ cup almond flour
- ¼ cup coconut four
- ¼ cup coconut flour
- ½ tsp. paprika
- ½ tsp. cumin
- 1 ½ tsp. chili pepper spice
- 1 tsp. onion powder
- ½ tsp. sunflower seeds
- 1 whole egg
- ¼ cup unsalted almond butter

Directions:

1. Preheat your oven to 350 F.
2. Line a baking sheet with parchment paper and keep it on the side. Add ingredients to your food processor and pulse until you have a nice dough.
3. Divide dough into two equal parts.
4. Place one ball on a sheet of parchment paper and cover with another sheet; roll it out. Cut into crackers and repeat with the other ball.
5. Transfer the prepped dough to a baking tray and bake for 8-10 min.
6. Remove from oven and serve. Enjoy!

58. DOLMAS WRAP

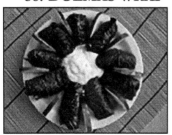

Preparation Time: 10 min.

Cooking Time: 10 min.

Servings: 2

Nutrition - Per Serving: Calories: 341

Fat 12.9; Fiber 9.2; Carbs 52.4; Protein 13.2

Phosphorus: 206mg; Potassium: 125mg; Sodium: 181mg

Ingredients:

- 2 whole wheat wraps
- 6 dolmans (stuffed grape leaves)
- 1 tomato, chopped
- 1 cucumber, chopped
- 2 oz Greek yogurt
- ½ tsp. minced garlic
- ¼ cup lettuce, chopped
- 2 oz Feta, crumbled

Directions:

1. The mixing bowl combines chopped tomato, cucumber, Greek yogurt, minced garlic, lettuce, and Feta.
2. When the mixture is homogenous transfer it in the center of every wheat wrap.
3. Arrange dolma over the vegetable mixture.
4. Carefully wrap the wheat wraps.

59. GREEN PALAK PANEER

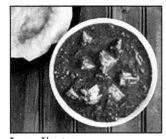

Preparation Time: 5 min.

Cooking Time: 10 min.

Servings: 4

Nutrition - Per Serving: Calories: 367

Fat: 26g; Carbs: 21g; Protein: 16g

Phosphorus: 236mg; Potassium: 385mg; Sodium: 128mg

Ingredients:

- 1-pound spinach
- 2 cups cubed paneer (vegan)
- 2 tbsp. coconut oil
- 1 tsp. cumin
- 1 chopped up onion
- 1-2 tsp. hot green chili minced up
- 1 tsp. minced garlic
- 15 cashews
- 4 tbsp. almond milk
- 1 tsp. Garam masala
- Flavored vinegar as needed

Directions:

1. Add cashews and milk to a blender and blend well.
2. Set your pot to Sauté mode and add coconut oil; allow the oil to heat up.
3. Add cumin seeds, garlic, green chilies, ginger and sauté for 1 min.
4. Add onion and sauté for 2 min.
5. Add chopped spinach, flavored vinegar and a cup of water.
6. Lock up the lid and cook on HIGH pressure for 10 min.
7. Quick-release the pressure.
8. Add ½ cup of water and blend to a paste.
9. Add cashew paste, paneer and Garam Masala and stir thoroughly.
10. Serve over hot rice!

60. SPORTY BABY CARROTS

Preparation Time: 5 min.   **Cooking Time:** 5 min.   **Servings**: 4

Ingredients:

- 1-pound baby carrots
- 1 cup water
- 1 tbsp. clarified ghee
- 1 tbsp. chopped up fresh mint leaves
- Sea flavored vinegar as needed

Directions:

1. Place a steamer rack on top of your pot and add the carrots.
2. Add water.
3. Lock the lid and cook at HIGH pressure for 2 min.
4. Do a quick release.
5. Pass the carrots through a strainer and drain them.
6. Wipe the insert clean.
7. Return the insert to the pot and set the pot to Sauté mode.
8. Add clarified butter and allow it to melt.
9. Add mint and sauté for 30 seconds.
10. Add carrots to the insert and sauté well.
11. Remove them and sprinkle with bit of flavored vinegar on top.

Nutrition - Per Serving: Calories: 131; Fat: 10g; Carbs: 11g; Protein: 1g; Phosphorus: 116mg; Potassium: 185mg; Sodium: 81mg

---

61. TRADITIONAL BLACK BEAN CHILI

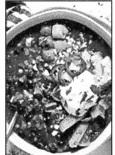

Preparation Time: 10 min.

Cooking Time: 4 hs

Servings: 4

Nutrition - Per Serving:

Calories: 211

Fat: 3g

Carbs: 22g

Protein: 5g

Phosphorus: 216mg

Potassium: 245mg

Sodium: 201mg

Ingredients:

- 1 ½ cups red bell pepper, chopped
- 1 cup yellow onion, chopped
- 1 ½ cups mushrooms, sliced
- 1 tbsp. olive oil
- 1 tbsp. chili powder
- 2 garlic cloves, minced
- 1 tsp. chipotle chili pepper, chopped
- ½ tsp. cumin, ground
- 16 ounces canned black beans, drained and rinsed
- 2 tbsp. cilantro, chopped
- 1 cup tomatoes, chopped

Directions:

1. Add red bell peppers, onion, dill, mushrooms, chili powder, garlic, chili pepper, cumin, black beans, and tomatoes to your Slow Cooker.
2. Stir well.
3. Place lid and cook on HIGH for 4 hs.
4. Sprinkle cilantro on top.
5. Serve and enjoy!

62. VERY WILD MUSHROOM PILAF

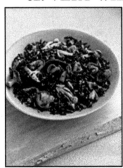

Preparation Time: 10 min.

Cooking Time: 3 hs

Servings: 4

Nutrition - Per Serving:

Calories: 210

Fat: 7g

Carbs: 16g

Protein: 4

Phosphorus: 266mg

Potassium: 232mg

Sodium: 176mg

Ingredients:

- 1 cup wild rice
- 2 garlic cloves, minced
- 6 green onions, chopped
- 2 tbsp. olive oil
- ½ pound baby Bella mushrooms
- 2 cups water

Directions:

1. Add rice, garlic, onion, oil, mushrooms and water to your Slow Cooker.
2. Stir well until mixed.
3. Place lid and cook on LOW for 3 hs.
4. Stir pilaf and divide between serving platters.
5. Enjoy!

63. CHILLED CHICKEN, ARTICHOKE AND ZUCCHINI PLATTER

Preparation Time: 10 min.   **Cooking Time:** 5 min.   **Servings**: 4

Ingredients:

- 2 medium chicken breasts, cooked and cut into 1-inch cubes
- ¼ cup extra virgin olive oil
- 2 cups artichoke hearts, drained and roughly chopped
- 3 large zucchinis, diced/cut into small rounds
- 1 can (15 ounce) chickpeas
- 1 cup Kalamata olives
- ½ tsp. Fresh ground black pepper
- ½ tsp. Italian seasoning
- ¼ cup parmesan, grated

Directions:

1. Take a large skillet and place it over medium heat, heat up olive oil.
2. Add zucchini and sauté for 5 min., season with salt and pepper.
3. Remove from heat and add all the listed ingredients to the skillet.
4. Stir until combined.
5. Transfer to glass container and store. Serve and enjoy!

Nutrition - Per Serving: Calories: 457; Fat: 22g; Carbs: 30g; Protein: 24g; Phosphorus: 216mg; Potassium: 285mg; Sodium: 157mg

64. CHICKEN AND CARROT STEW

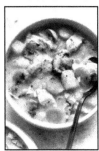

Preparation Time: 15 min.

Cooking Time: 6 hs

Servings: 6

Nutrition - Per Serving:

Calories: 182   Protein: 39g   Sodium: 212mg

Fat: 4g   Phosphorus: 216mg

Carbs: 10g   Potassium: 285mg

Ingredients:

- 4 chicken breasts, boneless and cubed
- 2 cups chicken broth
- 1 cup tomatoes, chopped
- 3 cups carrots, peeled and cubed
- 1 tsp. thyme dried
- 1 cup onion, chopped
- 2 garlic cloves, minced
- Pepper to taste

Directions:

1. Add all the ingredients to the Slow Cooker.
2. Stir and close the lid.
3. Cook for 6 hs.
4. Serve hot and enjoy!

65. TASTY SPINACH PIE

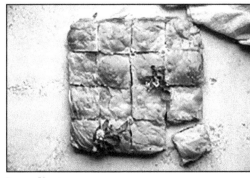

Preparation Time: 10 min.

Cooking Time: 4 hs

Servings: 2

Nutrition - Per Serving: Calories: 201

Fat: 6g

Carbs: 8g

Protein: 5g

Phosphorus: 216mg; Potassium: 275mg; Sodium: 121mg

Ingredients:

- 10 ounces spinach
- 2 cups baby Bella mushrooms, chopped
- 1 red bell pepper, chopped
- 1 ½ cups low-fat cheese, shredded
- 8 whole eggs
- 1 cup coconut cream
- 2 tbsp. chives, chopped
- Pinch of pepper
- ½ cup almond flour
- ¼ tsp. baking soda

Directions:

1. Take a bowl and add eggs, coconut cream, chives, pepper and whisk well.
2. Add almond flour, baking soda, cheese, mushrooms bell pepper, spinach and toss well.
3. Grease your cooker and transfer mix to the Slow Cooker.
4. Place lid and cook on LOW for 4 hs.
5. Slice and enjoy!

66. MESMERIZING CARROT AND PINEAPPLE MIX

Preparation Time: 10 min.   **Cooking Time:** 6 hs   **Servings**: 10

Ingredients:

- 1 cup raisins
- 6 cups water
- 23 ounces natural applesauce
- 2 tbsp. stevia
- 2 tbsp. cinnamon powder
- 14 ounces carrots, shredded
- 8 ounces canned pineapple, crushed
- 1 tbsp. pumpkin pie spice

Directions:

1. Add carrots, applesauce, raisins, stevia, cinnamon, pineapple, pumpkin pie spice to your Slow Cooker and gently stir.
2. Place lid and cook on LOW for 6 hs.
3. Serve and enjoy!

Nutrition - Per Serving: Calories: 179; Fat: 5g; Carbs: 15g; Protein: 4g; Phosphorus: 216mg; Potassium: 285mg; Sodium: 134mg

67. BLACKBERRY CHICKEN WINGS

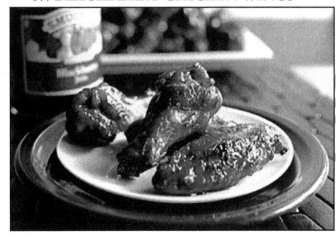

Preparation Time: 35 min.

Cooking Time: 50min.

Servings: 4

Nutrition - Per Serving:

Calories: 502

Fat: 39g

Carbs: 01.8g

Protein: 34g

Phosphorus: 216mg

Potassium: 305mg

Sodium: 131mg

Ingredients:

- 3 pounds chicken wings, about 20 pieces
- ½ cup blackberry chipotle jam
- Sunflower seeds and pepper to taste
- ½ cup water

Directions:

1. Add water and jam to a bowl and mix well. Place chicken wings in a zip bag and add two-thirds of the marinade.
2. Season with sunflower seeds and pepper.
3. Let it marinate for 30 min.
4. Pre-heat your oven to 400 F.
5. Prepare a baking sheet and wire rack, place chicken wings in wire rack and bake for 15 min.
6. Brush remaining marinade and bake for 30 min. more.
7. Enjoy!

68. HEALTHY CHICKEN CREAM SALAD

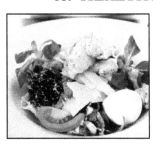

Preparation Time: 5 min.

Cooking Time: 50 min.

Servings: 3

Nutrition - Per Serving:

Calories: 415

Fat: 24g; Carbs: 4g; Protein: 40g

Phosphorus: 216mg; Potassium: 212mg; Sodium: 141mg

Ingredients:

- 2 chicken breasts
- 1 ½ cups low fat cream
- 3 ounces celery
- 2-ounce green pepper, chopped
- ½ ounce green onion, chopped
- ½ cup low fat mayo
- 3 hard-boiled eggs, chopped

Directions:

1. Pre-heat your oven to 350 F.
2. Take a baking sheet and place chicken, cover with cream. Bake for 30-40 min. Take a bowl and mix in the chopped celery, peppers, onions.
3. Chop the baked chicken into bite-sized portions. Peel and chop the hard-boiled eggs. Take a large salad bowl and mix in eggs, veggies and chicken.
4. Toss well and serve.

69. GENEROUSLY SMOTHERED PORK CHOPS

Preparation Time: 10 min.   **Cooking Time:** 30 min.   **Servings**: 4

Ingredients:

- 4 pork chops, bone-in
- 2 tbsp. of olive oil
- ¼ cup vegetable broth
- ½ pound Yukon gold potatoes, peeled and chopped
- 1 large onion, sliced
- 2 garlic cloves, minced
- 2 tsp. rubbed sage
- 1 tsp. thyme, ground
- Pepper as needed

Directions:

1. Pre-heat your oven to 350 F.
2. Take a large sized skillet and place it over medium heat. Add a tbsp. of oil and allow the oil to heat up. Add pork chops and cook them for 4-5 min. per side until browned. Transfer chops to a baking dish. Pour broth over the chops.
3. Add remaining oil to the pan and sauté potatoes, onion, garlic for 3-4 min.
4. Take a large bowl and add potatoes, garlic, onion, thyme, sage, pepper.
5. Transfer this mixture to the baking dish (wish pork). Bake for 20-30 min.
6. Serve and enjoy!

Nutrition - Per Serving: Calorie: 261, Fat: 10g, Carbs: 1.3g, Protein: 2g, Phosphorus: 196mg, Potassium: 285mg; Sodium: 111mg

70. SAUTEED CHICKPEA AND LENTIL MIX

Preparation Time: 10 min.   **Cooking Time:** 50 min.   **Servings:** 4

Ingredients:

- cup chickpeas, half-cooked
- cup lentils
- 5 cups chicken stock
- ½ cup fresh cilantro, chopped
- tsp. salt
- ½ tsp. chili flakes
- ¼ cup onion, diced
- tbsp. tomato paste

Directions:

1. Place chickpeas in the pan. Add water, salt, and chili flakes. Boil the chickpeas for 30 min. over the medium heat. Then add diced onion, lentils, and tomato paste. Stir well.
2. Close the lid and cook the mix for 15 min.
3. After this, add chopped cilantro, stir the meal well and cook it for 5 min. more.
4. Let the cooked lunch chill little before serving.

Nutrition: Calories 370 Fat 4.3 Fiber 23.7 Carbs 61.6 Protein 23.2 Phosphorus: 110mg Potassium: 117mg Sodium: 75mg

71. JAPANESE POTATO AND BEEF CROQUETTES

Preparation Time: 10 min.   **Cooking Time**: 20 min.   **Servings**: 10

Ingredients:

- 3 medium russet potatoes, peeled and chopped
- tbsp. almond butter
- tbsp. vegetable oil
- onions, diced
- ¾ pound ground beef
- tsp. light coconut aminos
- All-purpose flour for coating
- eggs, beaten
- Panko bread crumbs for coating
- ½ cup oil, frying

Directions:

1. Take a saucepan and place it over medium-high heat; add potatoes and sunflower seeds water, boil for 16 min.
2. Remove water and put potatoes in another bowl, add almond butter and mash the potatoes. Take a frying pan and place it over medium heat, add 1 tbsp. oil and let it heat up.
3. Add onions and stir fry until tender. Add coconut aminos to beef to onions.
4. Keep frying until beef is browned.
5. Mix the beef with the potatoes evenly.
6. Take another frying pan and place it over medium heat; add half a cup of oil.
7. Form croquettes using the mashed potato mixture and coat them with flour, then eggs and finally breadcrumbs.
8. Fry patties until golden on all sides.
9. Enjoy!

Nutrition: Calories: 239 Fat: 4g Carbs: 20g Protein: 10g Phosphorus: 120mg Potassium: 107mg Sodium: 75mg

72. TRADITIONAL BLACK BEAN CHILI

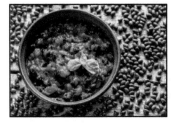

Preparation Time: 10 min.

Cooking Time: 4 hs

Servings: 4

Ingredients:

- ½ cups red bell pepper, chopped
- cup yellow onion, chopped
- ½ cups mushrooms, sliced
- tbsp. olive oil
- tbsp. chili powder
- garlic cloves, minced
- tsp. chipotle chili pepper, chopped
- ½ tsp. cumin, ground
- 16 ounces canned black beans, drained and rinsed
- tbsp. cilantro, chopped
- cup Red bell peppers, chopped

Directions:

1. Add red bell peppers, onion, dill, mushrooms, chili powder, garlic, chili pepper, cumin, black beans, and Red bell peppers to your Slow Cooker.
2. Stir well.
3. Place lid and cook on HIGH for 4 hs.
4. Sprinkle cilantro on top.
5. Serve and enjoy!

Nutrition: Calories: 211 Fat: 3g Carbs: 22g Protein: 5g Phosphorus: 90mg Potassium: 107mg Sodium: 75mg

73. LEMON ORZO SPRING SALAD

Preparation Time: 15 min.   **Cooking Time**: 10 min   **Servings** 4

Ingredients

- ¼ cup fresh, diced yellow peppers
- ¼ box or ¾ cup orzo pasta
- 1 tsp. lemon zest
- ¼ cup fresh, diced green peppers
- 2 cups medium-cubed, fresh zucchini
- ¼ cup fresh, diced red peppers
- 2 tbsp. chopped fresh rosemary
- 3 tbsp. fresh lemon juice
- ½ tsp. dried oregano
- ½ cup fresh, diced Vidalia or red onion
- ¼ cup and 2 tbsp. olive oil
- ½ tsp. black pepper
- 3 tbsp. Parmesan cheese, grated
- ½ tsp. red pepper flakes

Directions

1. Cook the orzo pasta, drain, and let sit according to the package instructions. (Not to rinse.)
2. On moderate heat, sauté the onions, zucchini, and peppers with 2 tbsp. of oil in a large mixing pan until translucent.
3. In a big bowl, add the lemon zest, lemon juice, half a cup of olive oil, rosemary, cheese, oregano, pepper, and red pepper flakes.
4. In a big bowl, add the orzo pasta and sautéed vegetables and fold gently till it's mixed.
5. Serve

Nutrition Per Serving: Calories 330 Protein 6 g Sodium 79 mg Phosphorus 134 mg Fiber 5 g Potassium 376 mg

74. SHRIMP NOODLE AND VEGGIE SALAD

Preparation Time: 10 min.   **Cooking Time**: 2 min   **Servings** 10

Ingredients

- 4 cups cooked, deveined, peeled, tailless, and cut in half cocktail shrimp; or 14-oz. pack of salad shrimp, cooked
- 1 lb. package of dry Spaghetti, chilled and cooked noodles (do not rinse)
- 2 cups broccoli florets (fresh)

Low-Sodium Soy Sauce Substitute (1 cup):

- 1 tsp. low-sodium soy sauce
- 4 tsp. low sodium Better Than Bouillon Chicken Base
- 1 cup scallions (fresh), sliced on the bias
- 2 cups fresh, chopped shitake mushrooms
- 2 tbsp. sesame oil
- 1 cup shredded, fresh carrots
- ½ cup rice wine vinegar
- 2 tsp. chili oil

- 2 tsp. dark molasses
- 4 tsp. Balsamic vinegar
- ¼ tsp. white pepper
- 1 tbsp. chopped, fresh ginger
- 2 tbsp. chopped, fresh garlic
- ¼ cup lime juice (2 limes), and zest of 1 lime (1 tbsp.)
- ¼ cup soy sauce substitute (low-sodium)

- ¼ tsp. ground ginger
- 1½ cups water
- ¼ tsp. garlic powder

Directions

1. Combine the substitute soy sauce ingredients in a small saucepan.
2. On medium flame, stir. Allow it to slightly thicken and reduce to around 1 cup. Store the rest in the fridge.
3. Then, in a big bowl, combine the ingredients together and set aside. Blend together the remaining ingredients in the blender until well mixed, around 1 min.
4. Pour the dressing mixture over the pasta mixture. Toss till it's covered well, then eat.

Nutrition Per Serving: Calories 254 Protein 13 g Sodium 433 mg Phosphorus 229 mg Fiber 3 g Potassium 325 mg

75. CHICKEN BROCCOLI NAPLES

Preparation Time: 30 min.   **Cooking Time**: 20 min   **Servings** 4

Ingredients

- 2 cups fresh, blanched broccoli florets
- 1 lb. pizza dough
- 1 cup low-salt, shredded mozzarella cheese
- 2 cups cooked chicken breast, diced
- 1 tbsp. chopped fresh oregano
- 1 tbsp. chopped fresh garlic
- 2 tbsp. flour
- 1 tsp. red pepper flakes, crushed

☞ 2 tbsp. olive oil

Directions

•

1. Preheat the oven to 400° F.
2. In a big bowl, mix the chicken, pepper flakes, cheese, garlic, oregano, broccoli and set aside.
3. Powder tabletop with flour and roll dough out until you hit a rectangular form of 11" x 14".
4. Place the chicken mixture along the longest line, about two inches from the side of the dough.
5. Pinch and roll the seam and ends till sealed tightly. Use olive oil to brush the top and make 3 tiny slits on the surface of the dough.
6. Bake on the lightly greased baking sheet tray for 8-12 min. or till golden brown.
7. Remove, give 3-5 min. to settle, then slice and serve.

Nutrition Per Serving: Calories 522 Protein 38 g Sodium 607 mg Phosphorus 400 mg Fiber 2.9 g Potassium 546 mg

76. CRISPY CUCUMBER SALAD

Preparation Time: 5 min.   **Cooking Time**: 0 min   **Servings** 4

Ingredients

☞ 2 tbsp. Caesar or Italian salad dressing
☞ 2 cups fresh cucumber, sliced into ¼-inch slices (peeling is optional)
☞ Ground black pepper (according to taste)

Directions

1. Combine the salad dressing and cucumber in a medium-size bowl with a lid.
2. Shake to coat after covering with a lid
3. Use ground black pepper to sprinkle. Refrigerate.
4. Serve

Nutrition Per Serving: Calories 27 Protein 0 g Sodium 74 mg Phosphorus 14 mg Fiber 0 g Potassium 90 mg

77. SAVORY AND SMOKY SALMON DIP

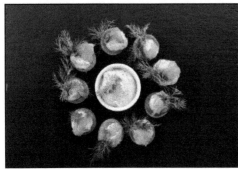

Preparation Time: 40 min.

Cooking Time: 6 min

Servings 12

Ingredients

☞ 2 tsp. smoked paprika
☞ 1 cup cream cheese
☞ ¼ cup capers
☞ Zest of half a lemon (1 tsp.) and ¼ cup lemon juice
☞ 2 tsp. finely diced, red onions
☞ 1 tsp. ground black pepper
☞ 1 tbsp. chopped, fresh parsley

☞ 1 lb. fresh boneless, skinless salmon (cut into 4 pieces)

Directions

1. For 4-6 min. on medium-high heat, scoop up the salmon in two cups of water and 1 tsp. of smoked paprika; the pot must be closed but should not hit a boil. Remove and chill for around 30 min.
2. Mix together all of the other ingredients till smooth. Split the salmon into bite-sized bits and fold them into a mixture of cream cheese.
3. Chill for 20-30 min., the salmon dip. Serve with carrots, celery sticks, corn chips or wrapped in an iceberg lettuce leaf.

Nutrition Per Serving: Calories 133 Protein 10 g Sodium 147 mg Phosphorus 110 mg Fiber 0 mg Potassium 259 mg

78. GREEN PALAK PANEER

Preparation Time: 5 min   **Cooking Time:** 10 min   **Servings**: 4

Ingredients:

- 1-pound green lettuce
- 2 cups cubed paneer (vegan)
- 2 tbsp. coconut oil
- tsp. cumin
- chopped up onion
- 1-2 tsp. hot green chili minced up
- tsp. minced garlic
- 15 cashews
- 4 tbsp. almond milk
- tsp. Garam masala
- Flavored vinegar as needed

Directions:

1. Add cashews and milk to a blender and blend well. Set your pot to Sauté mode and add coconut oil; allow the oil to heat up.
2. Add cumin seeds, garlic, green chilies, ginger and sauté for 1 min. Add onion and sauté for 2 min. Add chopped green lettuce, flavored vinegar and a cup of water.
3. Lock up the lid and cook on HIGH pressure for 10 min.
4. Quick release the pressure.
5. Add ½ cup of water and blend to a paste.
6. Add cashew paste, paneer and Garam Masala and stir thoroughly.
7. Serve over hot rice!

Nutrition: Calories: 367 Fat: 26g Carbs:21g Protein:16g Phosphorus:110mg Potassium:117mg Sodium:75mg

79. CUCUMBER SANDWICH

Preparation Time: 1 h   **Cooking Time**: 5 min   **Servings**: 2

Ingredients:

- 6 tsp. of cream cheese
- 1 pinch of dried dill weed
- 3 tsp. of mayonnaise
- .25 tsp. dry Italian dressing mix
- 4 slices of white bread
- .5 of a cucumber

Directions:

1. Prepare the cucumber and cut it into slices.
2. Mix cream cheese, mayonnaise, and Italian dressing. Chill for one h. Distribute the mixture onto the white bread slices.
3. Place cucumber slices on top and sprinkle with the dill weed.
4. Cut in halves and serve.

Nutrition: Calories: 143 Fat: 6g Carbs: 16.7g Protein: 4g Sodium: 255mg Potassium: 127mg Phosphorus: 64mg

80. PIZZA PITAS

Preparation Time: 10 min   **Cooking Time**: 10 min   **Servings**: 1

Ingredients:

- .33 cup of mozzarella cheese
- 2 pieces of pita bread, 6 inches in size
- 6 tsp. of chunky tomato sauce
- 2 cloves of garlic (minced)
- .25 cups of onion, chopped small
- .25 tsp. of red pepper flakes
- .25 cup of bell pepper, chopped small
- 2 ounces of ground pork, lean
- No-stick oil spray
- .5 tsp. of fennel seeds

Directions:

1. Preheat oven to 400.
2. Put the garlic, ground meat, pepper flakes, onion, and bell pepper in a pan. Sauté until cooked. Grease a flat baking pan and put pitas on it. Use the mixture to spread on the pita bread.
3. Spread one tbsp. of the tomato sauce and top with cheese.
4. Bake for five to eight min, until the cheese is bubbling.

Nutrition: Calories: 284 Fat: 10g Carbs: 34g Protein: 16g Sodium: 795mg Potassium: 706mg Phosphorus: 416mg

81. LETTUCE WRAPS WITH CHICKEN

Preparation Time: 10 min   **Cooking Time**: 15 min   **Servings:** 4

Ingredients:

- 8 lettuce leaves
- .25 cups of fresh cilantro
- .25 cups of mushroom
- 1 tsp. of five spices seasoning
- .25 cups of onion
- 6 tsp. of rice vinegar
- 2 tsp. of hoisin
- 6 tsp. of oil (canola)
- 3 tsp. of oil (sesame)
- 2 tsp. of garlic
- 2 scallions
- 8 ounces of cooked chicken breast

Directions:

1. Mince together the cooked chicken and the garlic. Chop up the onions, cilantro, mushrooms, and scallions.
2. Use a skillet overheat, combine chicken to all remaining ingredients, minus the lettuce leaves. Cook for fifteen min, stirring occasionally.
3. Place .25 cups of the mixture into each leaf of lettuce.
4. Wrap the lettuce around like a burrito and eat.

Nutrition: Calories: 84 Fat: 4g Carbs: 9g Protein: 5.9g Sodium: 618mg Potassium: 258mg Phosphorus: 64mg

82. TURKEY PINWHEELS

Preparation Time: 10 min   **Cooking Time**: 15 min   **Servings**: 6

Ingredients:

- 6 toothpicks
- 8 oz. of spring mix salad greens
- 1 ten-inch tortilla
- 2 ounces of thinly sliced deli turkey
- 9 tsp. of whipped cream cheese
- 1 roasted red bell pepper

Directions:

1. Cut the red bell pepper into ten strips about a quarter-inch thick.
2. Spread the whipped cream cheese on the tortilla evenly.
3. Add the salad greens to create a base layer and then lay the turkey on top of it.
4. Space out the red bell pepper strips on top of the turkey.
5. Tuck the end and begin rolling the tortilla inward. Use the toothpicks to hold the roll into place and cut it into six pieces.
6. Serve with the swirl facing upward.

Nutrition: Calories: 206 Fat: 9g Carbs: 21g Protein: 9g Sodium: 533mg Potassium: 145mg Phosphorus: 47mg

83. CHICKEN TACOS

Preparation Time: 5 min   **Cooking Time**: 20 min   **Servings:** 4

Ingredients:

- 8 corn tortillas
- 1.5 tsp. of Sodium-free taco seasoning
- 1 juiced lime
- .5 cups of cilantro
- 2 green onions, chopped
- 8 oz. of iceberg or romaine lettuce, shredded or chopped
- .25 cup of sour cream
- 1 pound of boneless and skinless chicken breast

Directions:

1. Cook chicken, by boiling, for twenty min. Shred or chop cooked chicken into fine bite-sized pieces. Mix the seasoning and lime juice with the chicken.
2. Put chicken mixture and lettuce in tortillas.
3. Top with the green onions, cilantro, and sour cream.

Nutrition: Calories: 260 Fat: 3g Carbs: 36g Protein: 23g Sodium: 922mg Potassium: 445mg Phosphorus: 357mg

84. SAVORY MUFFINS WITH PROTEIN

Preparation time: 15 min.   **Cooking time**: 35 min.   **Servings:** 12

1. *Ingredients:*
   - 2 cups corn flakes
   - ½ cup unfortified almond milk
   - 4 large eggs
   - 2 tbsp. olive oil
   - 1/2 cup almond milk
   - 1 medium white onion, sliced

- 1 cup plain Greek yogurt
- ¼ cup pecans, chopped
- 1 tbsp. mixed seasoning blend, e.g., Mrs. dash

Directions:

1. Pre-heat the oven at 350°F/180°C. Heat the olive oil in the pan. Sauté the onions with the pecans and seasoning blend for a couple of min.
2. Add the other ingredients and toss well.
3. Split the mixture into 12 small muffin cups (lightly greased) and bake for 30–35 min or until an inserted knife or toothpick is coming out clean. Serve warm or keep at room temperature for a couple of days.

Nutrition: Calories: 106.58kcal Carbs: 8.20g Protein: 4.77g Sodium: 51.91mg Potassium: 87.83mg Phosphorus: 49.41mg Dietary Fiber: 0.58g Fat: 5g

85. SUNNY PINEAPPLE BREAKFAST SMOOTHIE

Preparation time: 1 min.   **Cooking time**: 1 min.   **Servings:** 1

Ingredients:

- ½ cup frozen pineapple chunks
- 2/3 cup almond milk
- ½ tsp. ginger powder
- 1 tbsp. agave syrup

Directions:

1. Blend everything until smooth (around 30 seconds).
2. Transfer into a tall glass or Mason jar.
3. Serve and enjoy.

Nutrition: Calories: 186kcal Carbs: 43.7g Sodium: 130mg Potassium: 135mg Phosphorus: 18mg Dietary Fiber: 2.4g Fat: 2.3g Protein: 2.28g

86. TOFU AND MUSHROOM SCRAMBLE

Preparation time: 5 min.   **Cooking time**: 8 min.   **Servings**: 2

Ingredients:

- ½ cup sliced white mushrooms
- 1/3 cup medium-firm tofu, crumbled
- 1 tbsp. chopped shallots
- 1/3 tsp. turmeric
- 1 tsp. cumin
- 1/3 tsp. smoked paprika
- ½ tsp. garlic salt
- Pepper
- 3 tbsp. vegetable oil

Directions:

1. Heat the oil and sauté the sliced mushrooms in a frying pan with the shallots until softened (around 3–4 min) over medium to high heat.
2. Add the tofu pieces and toss in the spices and the garlic salt. Toss lightly until tofu and mushrooms are nicely combined. Serve warm.

Nutrition: Calories: 220kcal Carbs: 2.59g Sodium: 88mg Potassium: 133.5mg Phosphorus: 68.5mg Dietary Fiber: 1.7g Fat: 23.7g Protein: 3.2g

87. ITALIAN APPLE FRITTERS

Preparation time: 5 min.   **Cooking time**: 8 min.   **Servings**: 4

Ingredients:

- 2 large apples, seeded, peeled, and thickly sliced in circles
- 3 tbsp. cornflour
- ½ tsp. water
- 1 tsp. sugar
- 1 tsp. cinnamon
- Vegetable oil (for frying)
- Sprinkle of icing sugar or honey

Directions:

1. Combine the cornflour, water, and sugar in a small bowl to make your batter.
2. Deep the apple rounds into the corn flour mix.
3. Heat enough vegetable oil to cover half of the pan's surface over medium to high heat.
4. Add the apple rounds into the pan and cook until golden brown.
5. Transfer into a shallow dish with absorbing paper on top and sprinkle with cinnamon and icing sugar.

Nutrition: Calories: 183kcal Carbs: 17.9g Protein: 0.3g Sodium: 2g Potassium: 100mg Phosphorus: 12.5mg Dietary fiber: 1.4g Fat: 14.17g

88. TURKEY BREAKFAST SAUSAGE

Preparation time: 3 min.   **Cooking time**: 6 min.   **Servings**: 6

Ingredients:

- 1 pound lean ground turkey
- 1 tsp. fennel seed
- ¼ tsp. garlic powder
- ¼ tsp. onion powder
- ¼ tsp. salt
- 2 tbsp. vegetable oil
- Pepper

Directions:

1. Combine all the ingredients and apart from the vegetable oil in a mixing bowl.
2. Form into long and flat (around 4-inch-long) patties.
3. In a frying pan, heat the oil.
4. Cook for 3 min on each side. Repeat until you cook all the patties.
5. Serve warm.

Nutrition: Calories: 74kcal Carbs: 0.1g Protein: 7g Sodium: 121.9g Potassium: 89.5mg Phosphorus: 75mg Dietary fiber: 0g Fat: 5.16g

89. BLUEBERRY SMOOTHIE BOWL

Preparation time: 1 min.   **Cooking time**: 1 min.   **Servings**: 1

Ingredients:

- ½ cup frozen blueberries
- ½ cup vanilla-flavored almond milk
- 1 tbsp. agave syrup
- 1 tsp. chia seeds

Directions:

1. Combine everything except for the chia seeds in the blender until smooth. You should end up with a thick smoothie paste.
2. Transfer into a cereal bowl and top with chia seeds on top

Nutrition: Calories: 278.5kcal Carbs: 38.72g Protein: 1.3g Sodium: 76.33mg Potassium: 229.1mg Phosphorus: 59.2mg Dietary Fiber: 7.4g Fat: 6g

90. TUNA TWIST

Preparation Time: 10 min   **Cooking Time**: 30 min   **Servings**: 4

Ingredients:

- 1 can of unsalted or water packaged tuna, drained
- 6 tsp. of vinegar
- 5 cup of cooked peas
- 5 cup celery (chopped)
- 3 tsp. of dried dill weed
- 12 oz. cooked macaroni
- cup of mayonnaise

Directions:

1. Stir together the macaroni, vinegar, and mayonnaise together until blended and smooth.
2. Stir in remaining ingredients.
3. Chill before serving.

Nutrition: Calories: 290 Fat: 10g Carbs: 32g Protein: 16g Sodium: 307mg Potassium: 175mg Phosphorus: 111mg

91. CIABATTA ROLLS WITH CHICKEN PESTO

Preparation Time: 10 min   **Cooking Time**: 20 min   **Servings**: 2

Ingredients:

- 6 tsp. of Greek yogurt
- 6 tsp. of pesto
- 2 small ciabatta rolls
- 8 oz. of a shredded iceberg or romaine lettuce
- 8 oz. of cooked boneless and skinless chicken breast, shredded
- tsp. of pepper

Directions:

1. Combine the shredded chicken, pesto, pepper, and Greek yogurt in a medium-sized bowl.
2. Slice and toast the ciabatta rolls.
3. Divide the shredded chicken and pesto mixture in half and make sandwiches with the ciabatta rolls. Top with shredded lettuce if desired.

Nutrition: Calories: 374 Fat: 10g Carbs: 40g Protein: 30g Sodium: 522mg Potassium: 360mg Phosphorus: 84mg

92. MARINATED SHRIMP PASTA SALAD

Preparation Time: 15 min   **Cooking Time**: 5 hs   **Servings**: 1

Ingredients:

- 1/4 cup of honey
- 1/4 cup of balsamic vinegar
- 1/2 of an English cucumber, cubed
- 1/2 pound of fully cooked shrimp
- 15 baby carrots
- 1.5 cups of dime-sized cut cauliflower
- 4 stalks of celery, diced
- 1/2 large yellow bell pepper (diced)
- 1/2 red onion (diced)
- 1/2 large red bell pepper (diced)
- 12 ounces of uncooked tri-color pasta (cooked)
- 3/4 cup of olive oil
- 3 tsp. of mustard (Dijon)
- 1/2 tsp. of garlic (powder)
- 1/2 tsp. pepper

Directions:

1. Cut vegetables and put them in a bowl with the shrimp.
2. Whisk together the honey, balsamic vinegar, garlic powder, pepper, and Dijon mustard in a small bowl. While still whisking, slowly add the oil and whisk it all together.
3. Add the cooked pasta to the bowl with the shrimp and vegetables and mix it.
4. Toss the sauce to coat the pasta, shrimp, and vegetables evenly.
5. Cover and chill for a minimum of five hs before serving. Stir and serve while chilled.

Nutrition: Calories: 205 Fat: 13g Carbs: 10g Protein: 12g Sodium: 363mg Potassium: 156mg Phosphorus: 109mg

93. CHICKEN EGG ROLLS

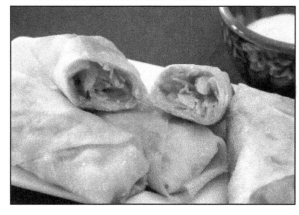

Preparation time: 10 min.
Cooking time: 12 min.
Servings: 14
Ingredients:

- 1 pound cooked chicken, diced
- 1/2 pound bean sprouts
- 1/2 pound cabbage, shredded
- 1 cup onion, chopped
- 2 tbsp. olive oil
- 1 tbsp. low-sodium soy sauce
- 1 garlic clove, minced
- 20 egg roll wrappers
- Oil for frying

Directions:

1. Add everything to a suitable bowl except for the roll wrappers. Mix these ingredients well to prepare the filling, then marinate for 30 min.
2. Place the roll wrappers on the working surface and divide the prepared filling on them. Fold the roll wrappers as per the package instructions and keep them aside.
3. Add oil to a deep wok and heat it to 350°F. Deep the egg rolls until golden brown on all sides.
4. Transfer the egg rolls to a plate lined with a paper towel to absorb all the excess oil. Serve warm.

Nutrition: Calories: 212kcal Total fat: 3.8g Saturated fat: 0.7g Cholesterol: 29mg Sodium: 329mg Carbs: 29g Dietary Fiber: 1.4g Sugars: 0.9g Protein: 14.9g Calcium: 37mg Phosphorous: 361mg Potassium: 171mg

CHAPTER 7. DINNER RECIPES

94. SEAFOOD CASSEROLE

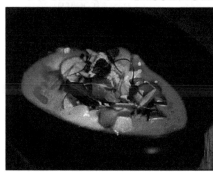

Preparation Time: 20 min.

Cooking Time: 45 min.

Servings: 6

Nutrition - Per Serving: Calories: 118

Fat: 4g

Carbs: 9g

Protein: 12g

Potassium: 199mg; Sodium: 235mg; Phosphorus: 102mg

Ingredients:

- 2 cups, peeled and diced into 1-inch pieces, Eggplant
- Butter, for greasing the baking dish
- 1 tbsp., Olive oil
- ½, chopped Sweet onion
- 1 tsp. Minced garlic
- 1, chopped Celery stalk
- ½, boiled and chopped Red bell pepper
- 3 tbsp., Freshly squeezed lemon juice
- 1 tsp. Hot sauce
- ¼ tsp. Creole seasoning mix
- ½ cup, uncooked, White rice
- 1 large Egg
- 4 ounces Cooked shrimp
- 6 ounces Queen crab meat

Directions:

1. Preheat the oven to 350F.
2. Boil the eggplant in a saucepan for 5 min. Drain and set aside.
3. Grease a 9-by-13-inch baking dish with butter and set aside. Heat the olive oil in a large skillet over medium heat.
4. Sauté the garlic, onion, celery, and bell pepper for 4 min. or until tender.
5. Add the sautéed vegetables to the eggplant, along with the lemon juice, hot sauce, seasoning, rice, and egg.
6. Stir to combine. Fold in the shrimp and crab meat. Spoon the casserole mixture into the casserole dish, patting down the top.
7. Bake for 25 to 30 min. or until casserole is heated through and rice is tender. Serve warm.

95. GROUND BEEF AND RICE SOUP

Preparation Time: 15 min.   **Cooking Time:** 40 min.   **Servings**: 6

Ingredients:

- ½ pound Extra-lean ground beef
- ½, chopped Small sweet onion
- 1 tsp. Minced garlic
- 2 cups Water
- 1 cup Low-sodium beef broth
- ½ cup, uncooked Long-grain white rice
- 1, chopped Celery stalk
- ½ cup, cut into – 1-inch pieces Fresh green beans
- 1 tsp. Chopped fresh thyme
- Ground black pepper

Directions:

1. Sauté the ground beef in a saucepan for 6 min. or until the beef is completely browned.
2. Drain off the excess fat and add the onion and garlic to the saucepan. Sauté the vegetables for about 3 min., or until they are softened. Add the celery, rice, beef broth, and water.
3. Bring the soup to a boil, reduce the heat to low and simmer for 30 min. or until the rice is tender. Add the green beans and thyme and simmer for 3 min.
4. Remove the soup from the heat and season with pepper.

Nutrition - Per Serving: Calories: 154; Fat: 7g; Carbs: 14g; Phosphorus: 76mg; Potassium: 179mg; Sodium: 133mg; Protein: 9g

96. COUSCOUS BURGERS

Preparation Time: 20 min   **Cooking Time:** 10 min.   **Servings**: 4

Ingredients:

- ½ cup, rinsed and drained Canned chickpeas
- 2 tbsp. Chopped fresh cilantro
- Chopped fresh parsley
- 1 tbsp. Lemon juice
- 2 tsp. Lemon zest
- 1 tsp. Minced garlic
- 2 ½ cups Cooked couscous
- 2 lightly beaten Eggs
- 2 tbsp. Olive oil

Directions:

1. Put the cilantro, chickpeas, parsley, lemon juice, lemon zest, and garlic in a food processor and pulse until a paste form. Transfer the chickpea mixture to a bowl and add the eggs and couscous. Mix well.
2. Chill the mixture in the refrigerator for 1 h. Form the couscous mixture into 4 patties. Heat olive oil in a skillet.
3. Place the patties in the skillet, 2 at a time, gently pressing them down with a spatula.
4. Cook for 5 min. or until golden and flip the patties over.
5. Cook the other side for 5 min. and transfer the cooked burgers to a plate covered with a paper towel.
6. Repeat with the remaining 2 burgers

Nutrition - Per Serving: Calories: 242; Fat: 10g; Carbs: 29g; Phosphorus: 108mg; Potassium: 168mg; Sodium: 43mg; Protein: 9g

97. BAKED FLOUNDER

Preparation Time: 20 min.   **Cooking Time:** 5 min.   **Servings**: 4

Ingredients:

- ¼ cup Homemade mayonnaise
- Juice of 1 lime
- Zest of 1 lime
- ½ cup Chopped fresh cilantro
- 4 (3-ounce) Flounder fillets
- Ground black pepper

Directions:

1. Preheat the oven to 400F.
2. In a bowl, stir together the cilantro, lime juice, lime zest, and mayonnaise.
3. Place 4 pieces of foil, about 8 by 8 inches square, on a clean work surface.

4. Place a flounder fillet in the center of each square.
5. Top the fillets evenly with the mayonnaise mixture. Season the flounder with pepper.
6. Fold the sides of the foil over the fish, creating a snug packet, and place the foil packets on a baking sheet. Bake the fish for 4 to 5 min.
7. Unfold the packets and serve.

Nutrition - Per Serving: Calories: 92; Fat: 4g; Carbs: 2g; Phosphorus: 208mg; Potassium: 137mg; Sodium: 267mg Protein: 12g

98. PERSIAN CHICKEN

Preparation Time: 10 min. **Cooking Time:** 20 min. **Servings**: 5

Ingredients:

- ½, chopped Sweet onion
- ¼ cup Lemon juice
- 1 tbsp. Dried oregano
- 1 tsp. Minced garlic
- 1 tsp. Sweet paprika
- ½ tsp. Ground cumin
- ½ cup Olive oil
- 5 Boneless, skinless chicken thighs

Directions:

1. Put the cumin, paprika, garlic, oregano, lemon juice, and onion in a food processor and pulse to mix the ingredients.
2. Keep the motor running and add the olive oil until the mixture is smooth.
3. Place the chicken thighs in a large sealable freezer bag and pour the marinade into the bag.
4. Seal the bag and place in the refrigerator, turning the bag twice, for 2 hs.
5. Remove the thighs from the marinade and discard the extra marinade.
6. Preheat the barbecue to medium.
7. Grill the chicken for about 20 min., turning once, until it reaches 165F.

Nutrition - Per Serving: Calories: 321; Fat: 21g; Carbs: 3g; Phosphorus: 131mg; Potassium: 220mg; Sodium: 86mg; Protein: 22g

99. PORK SOUVLAKI

Preparation Time: 20 min. **Cooking Time:** 12 min. **Servings**: 8

Ingredients:

- 3 tbsp. Olive oil
- 2 tbsp. Lemon juice
- 1 tsp. Minced garlic
- 1 tbsp. Chopped fresh oregano
- ¼ tsp. Ground black pepper
- 1 pound, cut in 2-inch cubes Pork leg

Directions:

1. In a bowl, stir together the lemon juice, olive oil, garlic, oregano, and pepper.
2. Add the pork cubes and toss to coat.
3. Place the bowl in the refrigerator, covered, for 2 hs to marinate. Thread the pork chunks onto 8 wooden skewers that have been soaked in water.
4. Preheat the barbecue to medium-high heat.
5. Grill the pork skewers for about 12 min., turning once, until just cooked through but still juicy.

Nutrition - Per Serving: Calories: 95; Fat: 4g; Carbs: 0g; Phosphorus: 125mg; Potassium: 230mg; Sodium: 29mg; Protein: 13g

100.   PORK MEATLOAF

Preparation Time: 10 min.   **Cooking Time:** 50 min.   **Servings**: 8

Ingredients:

- 1 pound 95% lean ground beef
- ½ cup Breadcrumbs
- ½ cup Chopped sweet onion
- 1 Egg
- 2 tbsp. Chopped fresh basil
- 1 tsp. Chopped fresh thyme
- 1 tsp. Chopped fresh parsley
- ¼ tsp. Ground black pepper
- 1 tbsp. Brown sugar
- 1 tsp. White vinegar
- ¼ tsp. Garlic powder

Directions:

1. Preheat the oven to 350F.
2. Mix the breadcrumbs, beef, onion, basil, egg, thyme, parsley, and pepper until well combined. Press the meat mixture into a 9-by-5-inch loaf pan.
3. In a small bowl, stir together the brown sugar, vinegar, and garlic powder.
4. Spread the brown sugar mixture evenly over the meat.
5. Bake the meatloaf for about 50 min. or until it is cooked through.
6. Let the meatloaf stand for 10 min. and then pour out any accumulated grease

Nutrition - Per Serving: Calories: 103; Fat: 3g; Carbs: 7g; Phosphorus: 112mg; Potassium: 190mg; Sodium: 87mg; Protein: 11g

101.   CHICKEN STEW

Preparation Time: 20 min.   **Cooking Time:** 50 min.   **Servings**: 6

Ingredients:

- 1 tbsp. Olive oil
- 1 pound, cut into 1-inch cubes Boneless, skinless chicken thighs
- ½, chopped Sweet onion
- 1 tbsp. Minced garlic
- 2 cups Chicken stock
- 1 cup, plus 2 tbsp. Water
- 1, sliced Carrot
- 2 stalks, sliced Celery
- 1, sliced thin Turnip
- 1 tbsp. Chopped fresh thyme
- 1 tsp. Chopped fresh rosemary
- 2 tsp. Cornstarch
- Ground black pepper to taste

Directions:

1. Place a large saucepan on medium heat and add the olive oil. Sauté the chicken for 6 min. or until it is lightly browned, stirring often.
2. Add the onion and garlic, and sauté for 3 min. Add 1-cup water, chicken stock, carrot, celery, and turnip and bring the stew to a boil.
3. Reduce the heat to low and simmer for 30 min. or until the chicken is cooked through and tender.
4. Add the thyme and rosemary and simmer for 3 min. more.
5. In a small bowl, stir together the 2 tbsp. of water and the cornstarch, add the mixture to the stew.
6. Stir to incorporate the cornstarch mixture and cook for 3 to 4 min. or until the stew thickens.
7. Remove from the heat and season with pepper.

Nutrition - Per Serving: Calories: 14; Fat: 8g; Carbs: 5g; Phosphorus: 53mg; Potassium: 192mg; Sodium: 214mg; Protein: 9g

102. BEEF CHILI

Preparation Time: 10 min.   **Cooking Time:** 30 min.   **Servings**: 2

Ingredients:

- 1, diced Onion
- 1, diced Red bell pepper
- 2 cloves, minced Garlic
- 6 oz Lean ground beef
- 1 tsp. Chili powder
- 1 tsp. Oregano
- 2 tbsp. Extra virgin olive oil
- 1 cup Water
- 1 cup Brown rice
- 1 tbsp. to serve Fresh cilantro

Directions:

1. Soak vegetables in warm water.
2. Bring a pan of water to the boil and add rice for 20 min.
3. Meanwhile, add the oil to a pan and heat on medium-high heat.
4. Add the pepper, onions, and garlic and sauté for 5 min. until soft. Remove and set aside. Add the beef to the pan and stir until browned.
5. Add the vegetables back into the pan and stir.
6. Now add the chili powder and herbs and the water, cover and turn the heat down a little to simmer for 15 min.
7. Meanwhile, drain the water from the rice, and the lid and steam while the chili is cooking. Serve hot with the fresh cilantro sprinkled over the top.

Nutrition - Per Serving: Calories: 459; Fat: 22g; Carbs: 36g; Phosphorus: 332mg; Potassium: 360mg; Sodium: 33mg; Protein: 22g

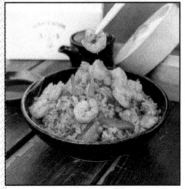

103. SHRIMP PAELLA

Preparation Time: 5 min.

Cooking Time: 10 min.

Servings: 2

Nutrition - Per Serving:

Calories: 221   Sodium 235 mg

Protein 17 g   Potassium 176 mg

Carbs 31 g   Phosphorus 189 mg

Fat 8 g

Ingredients:

- 1 cup cooked brown rice
- 1 chopped red onion
- 1 tsp. paprika
- 1 chopped garlic clove
- 1 tbsp. olive oil
- 6 oz. frozen cooked shrimp
- 1 deseeded and sliced chili pepper
- 1 tbsp. oregano

Directions:

1. Heat the olive oil in a large pan on medium-high heat. Add the onion and garlic and sauté for 2-3 min. until soft.
2. Now add the shrimp and sauté for a further 5 min. or until hot through.
3. Now add the herbs, spices, chili and rice with 1/2 cup boiling water.
4. Stir until everything is warm and the water has been absorbed.
5. Plate up and serve.

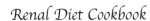

104.   SALMON & PESTO SALAD

Preparation Time:5 min.   **Cooking Time:**15 min.   **Servings:**2

Ingredients:

FOR THE PESTO:

- 1 minced garlic clove
- ½ cup fresh arugula
- ¼ cup extra virgin olive oi l
- ½ cup fresh basil

- 1 tsp.. black pepper

FOR THE SALMON:

- 4 oz. skinless salmon fillet
- 1 tbsp. coconut oil
- For the salad:

- ½ juiced lemon
- 2 sliced radishes
- ½ cup iceberg lettuce
- 1 tsp.. black pepper

Directions:

1. Prepare the pesto by blending all the ingredients for the pesto in a food processor or by grinding with a pestle and mortar. Set aside.
2. Add a skillet to the stove on medium-high heat and melt the coconut oil.
3. Add the salmon to the pan.
4. Cook for 7-8 min. and turn over.
5. Cook for a further 3-4 min. or until cooked through.
6. Remove fillets from the skillet and allow to rest.
7. Mix the lettuce and the radishes and squeeze over the juice of ½ lemon.
8. Flake the salmon with a fork and mix through the salad.
9. Toss to coat and sprinkle with a little black pepper to serve.

Nutrition - Per Serving: Calories: 221, Protein 13 g, Carbs 1 g, Fat 34 g, Sodium 80 mg, Potassium 119 mg, Phosphorus 158 mg

---

105.   BAKED FENNEL & GARLIC SEA BASS

Preparation Time:5 min.   **Cooking Time:**15 min.   **Servings:**2

Ingredients:

- 1 lemon
- ½ sliced fennel bulb

- 6 oz. sea bass fillets
- 1 tsp.. black pepper

- 2 garlic cloves

Directions:

1. Preheat the oven to 375°F/Gas Mark 5.
2. Sprinkle black pepper over the Sea Bass.
3. Slice the fennel bulb and garlic cloves.
4. Add 1 salmon fillet and half the fennel and garlic to one sheet of baking paper or tin foil.
5. Squeeze in 1/2 lemon juices.
6. Repeat for the other fillet.
7. Fold and add to the oven for 12-15 min. or until fish is thoroughly cooked through.
8. Meanwhile, add boiling water to your couscous, cover and allow to steam.
9. Serve with your choice of rice or salad.

Nutrition - Per Serving: Calories: 221, Protein 14 g, Carbs 3 g, Fat 2 g, Sodium 119 mg, Potassium 398 mg, Phosphorus 149 mg

---

106.   LEMON, GARLIC & CILANTRO TUNA AND RICE

Preparation Time:5 min.   **Cooking Time:**0 min.   **Servings:**2

Ingredients:

- ½ cup arugula
- 1 tbsp. extra-virgin olive oil
- 1 cup cooked rice
- 1 tsp.. black pepper

- ¼ finely diced red onion
- 1 juiced lemon
- 3 oz. canned tuna
- 2 tbsp. Chopped fresh cilantro

Directions:

1. Mix the olive oil, pepper, cilantro and red onion in a bowl.
2. Stir in the tuna, cover and leave in the fridge for as long as possible (if you can) or serve immediately.
3. When ready to eat, serve up with the cooked rice and arugula!

Nutrition - Per Serving: Calories: 221, Protein 11 g, Carbs 26 g, Fat 7 g, Sodium 143 mg, Potassium 197 mg, Phosphorus 182 mg

107. COD & GREEN BEAN RISOTTO

Preparation Time:4 min.   **Cooking Time:**40 min.   **Servings:**2

Ingredients:

- ½ cup arugula
- 1 finely diced white onion
- 4 oz. c od fillet
- 1 cup white rice
- 2 lemon wedges
- 1 cup boiling water
- ¼ tsp.. black pepper
- 1 cup low sodium chicken broth
- 1 tbsp. extra-virgin olive oil
- ½ cup green beans

Directions:

1. Heat the oil in a large pan on medium heat.
2. Sauté the chopped onion for 5 min. until soft before adding in the rice and stirring for 1-2 min. Combine the broth with boiling water.
3. Add half of the liquid to the pan and stir slowly.
4. Slowly add the rest of the liquid while continuously stirring for up to 20-30 min.
5. Stir in the green beans to the risotto.
6. Place the fish on top of the rice, cover and steam for 10 min. Ensure the water does not dry out and keep topping up until the rice is cooked thoroughly. Use your fork to break up the fish fillets and stir into the rice.
7. Sprinkle with freshly ground pepper to serve and a squeeze of fresh lemon.
8. Garnish with the lemon wedges and serve with the arugula.

Nutrition - Per Serving: Calories: 221, Protein 12 g, Carbs 29 g, Fat 8 g, Sodium 398 mg, Potassium 347 mg, Phosphorus 241 mg

108. SARDINE FISH CAKES

Preparation Time: 10 min.   **Cooking Time:** 10 min.   **Servings:**4

Ingredients:

- 11 oz sardines, canned, drained
- 1/3 cup shallot, chopped
- 1 tsp. chili flakes
- ½ tsp. salt
- 2 tbsp. wheat flour, whole grain
- 1 egg, beaten
- 1 tbsp. chives, chopped
- 1 tsp. olive oil
- 1 tsp. butter

Directions:

1. Put the butter in the skillet and melt it.
2. Add shallot and cook it until translucent.
3. After this, transfer the shallot in the mixing bowl.
4. Add sardines, chili flakes, salt, flour, egg, chives, and mix up until smooth with the help of the fork.
5. Make the medium size cakes and place them in the skillet.
6. Add olive oil.
7. Roast the fish cakes for 3 min. from each side over the medium heat.
8. Dry the cooked fish cakes with the paper towel if needed and transfer in the serving plates.

Nutrition - Per Serving: Calories: 221, Fat: 12.2g, Fiber: 0.1g, Carbs: 5.4g, Protein: 21.3g, Sodium: 708mg, Potassium: 376mg

109. CAJUN CATFISH

Preparation Time: 10 min. **Cooking Time:** 10 min. **Servings:**4

Ingredients:

- 16 oz catfish steaks (4 oz each fish steak)
- 1 tbsp. Cajun spices
- 1 egg, beaten
- 1 tbsp. sunflower oil

Directions:

1. Pour sunflower oil in the skillet and preheat it until shimmering.
2. Meanwhile, dip every catfish steak in the beaten egg and coat in Cajun spices.
3. Place the fish steaks in the hot oil and roast them for 4 min. from each side.
4. The cooked catfish steaks should have a light brown crust.

Nutrition - Per Serving: Calories: 263, Fat: 16.7g, Fiber: 0g, Carbs: 0.1g, Protein: 26.3g Sodium: 413mg, Potassium: 15mg

110. 4-INGREDIENTS SALMON FILLET

Preparation Time: 5 min. **Cooking Time:** 25 min. **Servings:**4

Ingredients:

- 4 oz salmon fillet
- ½ tsp. salt
- 1 tsp. sesame oil
- ½ tsp. sage

Directions:

1. Rub the fillet with salt and sage.
2. Place the fish in the tray and sprinkle it with sesame oil.
3. Cook the fish for 25 min. at 365F.
4. Flip the fish carefully onto another side after 12 min. of cooking.

Nutrition - Per Serving: Calories: 191, Fat: 11.6g, Fiber: 0.1g, Carbs: 0.2g, Protein: 22g, Sodium: 303mg, Potassium: 110mg

111. SPANISH COD IN SAUCE

Preparation Time: 10 min. **Cooking Time:** 5.5 hs **Servings:**2

Ingredients:

- 1 tsp. tomato paste
- 1 tsp. garlic, diced
- 1 white onion, sliced
- 1 jalapeno pepper, chopped
- 1/3 cup chicken stock
- 7 oz Spanish cod fillet
- 1 tsp. paprika
- 1 tsp. salt

Directions:

1. Pour chicken stock in the saucepan.
2. Add tomato paste and mix up the liquid until homogenous. Add garlic, onion, jalapeno pepper, paprika, and salt. Bring the liquid to boil and then simmer it. Chop the cod fillet and add it in the tomato liquid.
3. Close the lid and simmer the fish for 10 min. over the low heat.
4. Serve the fish in the bowls with tomato sauce.

Nutrition - Per Serving: Calories: 113, Fat: 1.2g, Fiber: 1.9g, Carbs: 7.2g, Protein: 18.9g; Sodium: 1528mg, Potassium: 881mg

112. FISH SHAKSHUKA

Preparation Time: 5 min.   **Cooking Time:** 15 min.   **Servings:**5

Ingredients:

- 5 eggs
- 1 cup tomatoes, chopped
- 3 bell peppers, chopped
- 1 tbsp. butter
- 1 tsp. tomato paste
- 1 tsp. chili pepper
- 1 tsp. salt
- 1 tbsp. fresh dill
- 5 oz cod fillet, chopped
- 1 tbsp. scallions, chopped

Directions:

1. Melt butter in the skillet and add chili pepper, bell peppers, and tomatoes.
2. Sprinkle the vegetables with scallions, dill, salt, and chili pepper. Simmer them for 5 min.
3. After this, add chopped cod fillet and mix up well.
4. Close the lid and simmer the ingredients for 5 min. over the medium heat.
5. Then crack the eggs over fish and close the lid.
6. Cook shakshuka with the closed lid for 5 min.

Nutrition - Per Serving: Calories: 143, Fat: 7.3g, Fiber: 1.6g, Carbs: 7.9g, Protein: 12.8g, Sodium 570mg, Potassium 317mg

113. BEEF KABOBS WITH PEPPER

Preparation Time: 5 Min.   **Cooking Time**: 10 Min.   **Servings**: 8

Ingredients:

- Pound of beef sirloin
- 1/2 Cup of vinegar
- tbsp. of salad oil
- Medium, chopped onion
- tbsp. of chopped fresh parsley
- 1/4 tsp. of black pepper
- Cut into strips green peppers

Directions:

1. Trim the fat from the meat; then cut it into cubes of 1 and 1/2 inches each
2. Mix the vinegar, the oil, the onion, the parsley and the pepper in a bowl
3. Place the meat in the marinade and set it aside for about 2 hs; make sure to stir from time to time.
4. Remove the meat from the marinade and alternate it on skewers instead with green pepper
5. Brush the pepper with the marinade and broil for about 10 min. 4 inches from the heat
6. Serve and enjoy your kabobs

Nutrition: Calories: 357 Total Fat: 24 g Saturated Fat: 0 g Cholesterol: 9 mg Sodium: 60 mg Carb: 0 g

114. BEEF ROAST

Preparation Time: 10 min.   **Cooking Time**: 75 min.   **Servings**: 4

Ingredients:

- 3 1/2 pounds beef roast
- 4 ounces mushrooms, sliced
- 12 ounces beef stock
- 1-ounce onion soup mix
- 1/2 cup Italian dressing

Directions:

1. Take a bowl and add the stock, onion soup mix, and Italian dressing. Then, stir.
2. Put beef roast in pan
3. Add the mushrooms and stock mix to the pan and cover with foil
4. Preheat your oven to 300 °F
5. Bake for 1 h and 15 min.
6. Let the roast cool
7. Slice and serve
8. Enjoy the gravy on top!

Nutrition: Calories: 700 Total Fat: 56 g Saturated Fat: 0 g Cholesterol: 0 mg Sodium: 0 mg Carb: 10 g

115. CALIFORNIA PORK CHOPS

Preparation Time: 10 min.   **Cooking Time**: 10 min.   **Servings**: 2

Ingredients:

- tbsp. fresh cilantro, chopped
- 1/2 cup chives, chopped

- large green bell peppers, chopped
- lb. 1" thick boneless pork chops
- tbsp. fresh lime juice
- cups cooked rice
- 1/8 tsp. dried oregano leaves
- 1/4 tsp. ground black pepper
- 1/4 tsp. ground cumin
- tbsp. butter
- lime

Directions:
1. Start by seasoning the pork chops with lime juice and cilantro.
2. Place them in a shallow dish.
3. Toss the chives with pepper, cumin, butter, oregano and rice in a bowl.
4. Stuff the bell peppers with this mixture and place them around the pork chops.
5. Cover the chop and bell peppers with a foil sheet and bake them for 10 min. in the oven at 375 F. Serve warm.

Nutrition: Calories: 265 Fat: 15g Saturated Fat: 0 g Cholesterol: 86 mg Sodium:70 mg Carbs:24 g Fiber: 1g Protein: 34g

116. CARIBBEAN TURKEY CURRY

Preparation Time: 10 min.   **Cooking Time**: 1 h 30 min.   **Servings**: 6

Ingredients:
- 3 1/2 lbs. turkey breast, with skin
- 1/4 cup butter, melted
- 1/4 cup honey
- tbsp. mustard
- tsp. curry powder
- tsp. garlic powder

Directions:
1. Place the turkey breast in a shallow roasting pan. Insert a meat thermometer to monitor the temperature.
2. Bake the turkey for 1.5 hs at 350 F until its internal temperature reaches 170 F.
3. Meanwhile, thoroughly mix honey, butter, curry powder, garlic powder, and mustard in a bowl.
4. Glaze the cooked turkey with this mixture liberally. Let it sit for 15 min. for absorption.
5. Slice and serve.

Nutrition: Calories: 275 Total Fat: 13 g Saturated Fat: 0 g Cholesterol: 82 mg Sodium: 122 mg Carbs: 90 g

117. CHICKEN FAJITAS

Preparation Time: 10 min.   **Cooking Time**: 10 min.   **Servings**: 8

Ingredients:
- 8 flour tortillas, 6" size
- 1/4 cup green pepper, cut in strips
- 1/4 cup red pepper, cut in strips
- 1/2 cup onion, sliced
- 1/2 cup cilantro
- 2 tbsp. canola oil
- 12 oz. boneless chicken breasts
- 1/4 tsp. black pepper
- 2 tsp. chili powder
- 1/2 tsp. cumin
- 2 tbsp. lemon juice

Directions:
1. Start by wrapping the tortillas in a foil.
2. Warm them up for 10 min. in a preheated oven at 300 F. Add oil to a nonstick pan.
3. Add lemon juice chicken and seasoning
4. Stir fry for 5 min. then add onion and peppers.
5. Continue cooking for 5 min. or until chicken is tender.
6. Stir in cilantro, mix well and serve in tortillas.

Nutrition: Calories: 343 Total Fat: 13 g Saturated Fat: 0 g Cholesterol: 53 mg Sodium: 281 mg Carb: 33 g

118. CHICKEN JULIEN

Preparation Time: 10 min.   **Cooking Time**: 10 min.   **Servings**: 4

Ingredients:
- 2 boneless skinless chicken breasts
- 1/2 shallot, chopped
- 2 tbsp. butter
- 2 tbsp. dry white wine
- 2 tbsp. chicken broth
- 1/2 cup green grapes, halved
- 1 tsp. dried tarragon
- 1/4 cup cream

Directions:
1. Place an 8-inch skillet over medium heat and add butter to melt.
2. Sear the chicken in the melted butter until golden-brown on both sides. Place the boneless chicken on a plate and set it aside.

Renal Diet Cookbook

3. Add shallot to the same skillet and stir until soft. Whisk cornstarch with broth and wine in a small bowl.
4. Pour this slurry into the skillet and mix well.
5. Place the chicken in the skillet and cook it on a simmer for 6 min.

6. Transfer the chicken to the serving plate.
7. Add cream, tarragon, and grapes.
8. Cook for 1 min., and then pour this sauce over the chicken.
9. Serve.

Nutrition: Calories: 306 Total Fat: 18 g Saturated Fat: 0 g Cholesterol: 124 mg Sodium: 167 mg Carbs: 9 g

119. CHICKEN AND APPLE CURRY

Preparation Time: 10 min **Cooking Time**: 1 h and 11 min **Servings**: 8

Ingredients:
- 8 boneless skinless chicken breasts
- 1/4 tsp. black pepper
- 2 medium apples, peeled, cored, and chopped
- 2 small onions, chopped
- garlic clove, minced
- tbsp. butter
- tbsp. curry powder
- 1/2 tbsp. dried basil
- tbsp. flour
- cup chicken broth
- cup of rice milk

Directions:
1. Preheat oven to 350°F.
2. Set the chicken breasts in a baking pan and sprinkle black pepper over it.
3. Place a suitably-sized saucepan over medium heat and add butter to melt.
4. Add onion, garlic, and apple, then sauté until soft.
5. Stir in basil and curry powder, and then cook for 1 min. Add flour and continue mixing for 1 min. Stir in rice milk and chicken broth, then stir cook for 5 min.
6. Pour this sauce over the chicken breasts in the baking pan. Bake the chicken for 60 min then serve.

Nutrition: Calories: 232 kcal Total Fat: 8 g Saturated Fat: 0 g Cholesterol: 85 mg Sodium: 118 mg Total Carbs: 11 g

120. LONDON BROIL

Preparation Time: 10 min **Cooking Time**: 5 min **Servings**: 4

Ingredients:
- 2 pounds flank steak
- 1/4 tsp. meat tenderizer
- 1 tbsp. sugar
- 2 tbsp. lemon juice
- 2 tbsp. soy sauce
- 1 tbsp. honey
- 1 tsp. herb seasoning blend

Directions:
1. Pound the meat with a mallet then place it in a shallow dish. Sprinkle meat tenderizer over the meat. Whisk rest of the ingredients and spread this marinade over the meat.
2. Marinate the meat for 4 hs in the refrigerator.
3. Bake the meat for 5 min per side at 350°F.
4. Slice and serve.

Nutrition: Calories: 184 kcal Total Fat: 8 g Saturated Fat: 0 g Cholesterol: 43 mg Sodium: 208 mg Total Carbs: 3 g

121. SLOW-COOKED BBQ BEEF

Preparation Time: 10 min **Cooking Time**: 30 min **Servings**: 4

Ingredients:
- 4-pound pot roast
- 2 cups of water
- ¾ cup ketchup
- 1/4 cup brown sugar
- 1/3 cup vinegar
- 1/2 tsp. allspice
- 1/4 cup onion

Directions:
1. Add 2 cups water and roast to a Crockpot and cover it.
2. Cook for 10 h on LOW setting, then drain it while keeping 1 cup of its liquid.
3. Transfer the cooked meat to a 9x13 pan and set it aside.
4. Whisk 1 cup liquid, ketchup, vinegar, brown sugar, minced onion, and allspice in a bowl.
5. Add beef to the marinade and mix well to coat, then marinate overnight in the refrigerator.
6. Spread it on a baking pan then bake for 30 min at 350°F. Serve.

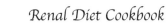

Nutrition: Calories: 303 kcal Total Fat: 17 g Saturated Fat: 0 g Cholesterol: 71 mg Sodium: 207 mg Total Carbs: 7 g

122. LEMON SPROUTS

Preparation Time: 10 min   **Cooking Time**: 0   **Servings**: 4

Ingredients:

- 1 pound Brussels sprouts, trimmed and shredded
- 8 tbsp. olive oil
- 1 lemon, juiced and zested
- Salt and pepper to taste
- ¾ cup spicy almond and seed mix

Directions:

1. Take a bowl and mix in lemon juice, salt, pepper and olive oil. Mix well
2. Stir in shredded Brussels sprouts and toss
3. Let it sit for 10 min
4. Add nuts and toss
5. Serve and enjoy!

Nutrition: Calories: 382 Fat: 36g Carbs: 9g Protein: 7g

123. LEMON AND BROCCOLI PLATTER

Preparation Time: 10 min   **Cooking Time**: 15 min   **Servings**: 6

Ingredients:

- 2 heads broccoli, separated into florets
- 2 tsp. extra virgin olive oil
- tsp. salt
- 1/2 tsp. black pepper
- garlic clove, minced
- 1/2 tsp. lemon juice

Directions:

1. Preheat your oven to 400 °F
2. Take a large-sized bowl and add broccoli florets
3. Drizzle olive oil and season with pepper, salt, and garlic
4. Spread the broccoli out in a single even layer on a baking sheet
5. Bake for 15-20 min until fork tender
6. Squeeze lemon juice on top
7. Serve and enjoy!

Nutrition: Calories: 49 Fat: 1.9g Carbs: 7g Protein: 3g

124. PORK BREAD CASSEROLE

Preparation time: 20 mins.   **Cooking time**: 55 mins.   **Servings**: 8

Ingredients:

- 2 tbsp. butter
- 1 pound pork sausage
- 1 yellow onion, chopped
- 18 slices white bread, cut into cubes
- 2 ½ cups sharp Cheddar cheese, grated
- 1/2 cup fresh parsley, chopped
- 6 large eggs
- 2 cups half-and-half cream
- 1 tsp. garlic powder
- 1/4 tsp. black pepper

Directions:

1. Switch on your gas oven and pre-heat it at 325°F. Layer a 9x9 inches casserole dish with bread cubes. Set a suitable-sized skillet over medium-high heat, then crumb the sausage in it. Cook the sausage until golden brown, then keep it aside.
2. Blend the eggs with the remaining ingredients in a blender until smooth. Stir in the sausage and spread this mixture over the bread pieces.
3. Bake the bread casserole for 55 minapproximately in the pre-heated oven.
4. Slice and serve.

Nutrition: Calories: 366kcal Total Fat: 26.4g Saturated Fat: 15.1g Cholesterol: 208mg Sodium: 436mg Carbs: 15.2g Dietary Fiber: 0.9g Sugars: 2.1g Protein: 17.5g Calcium: 378mg Phosphorous: 501 mg Potassium: 231mg

125. MEXICAN STYLE BURRITOS

Preparation time: 5 mins.   **Cooking time**: 15 mins.   **Servings**: 2

Ingredients

- 1 tbsp. olive oil
- 2 corn tortillas
- ¼ cup red onion, chopped
- ¼ cup red bell peppers, chopped
- ½ red chili, deseeded and chopped

🏴 2 eggs   🏴 Juice of 1 lime   🏴 1 tbsp. cilantro, chopped

Directions:

1. Turn the broiler to medium heat.
2. Place the tortillas underneath for 1 to 2 min on each side or until lightly toasted. Remove and keep the broiler on.
3. On a skillet, heat the oil and sauté the onion, chili and bell peppers for 5 to 6 min or until soft.
4. Pour eggs over the onions and peppers.
5. Place skillet under the broiler for 5 min or until the eggs are cooked.
6. Serve half the eggs and vegetables on top of each tortilla and sprinkle with cilantro and lime juice to serve.

Nutrition: Calories: 202kcal Fat: 13g Carb: 19g Phosphorus: 184mg Potassium: 233mg Sodium: 77mg Protein: 9g

126.   BLUEBERRY MUFFINS

Preparation time: 15 mins.   **Cooking time**: 30 mins.   **Servings**: 12

Ingredients:

🏴 2 cups unsweetened rice milk
🏴 1 tbsp. apple cider vinegar
🏴 3 ½ cups all-purpose flour
🏴 1 cup granulated sugar

🏴 1 tbsp. baking soda substitute
🏴 1 tsp. ground cinnamon
🏴 ½ tsp. ground nutmeg
🏴 Pinch ground ginger

🏴 ½ cup canola oil
🏴 2 tbsp. pure vanilla extract
🏴 2 ½ cups fresh blueberries

Directions:

1. Preheat the oven to 375°F.
2. Arrange the cups of a muffin pan thru paper liners. Set aside.
3. In a small bowl, put the rice milk and vinegar.
4. Set aside for 10 mins.
5. In a large bowl, stir together the sugar, flour, baking soda, nutmeg, cinnamon, ginger, and wait until it is well mixed.
6. Add the vanilla and oil to the milk mixture and stir to blend. Add the milk combination to the dry fixings and stir until just combined.
7. Fold in the blueberries. Spoon the muffin batter squarely into the cups.
8. Bake the muffins for 30 min or until golden. Cool for 15 min and serve.

Nutrition: Calories: 331kcal Fat: 11g Carb: 52g Phosphorus: 90mg Potassium: 89mg Sodium: 35mg Protein: 6g

127.   CHICKEN LIVER STEW

Preparation Time: 10 min   **Cooking Time**: 20 min   **Servings**: 2

Ingredients:

🏴 10 ounces chicken livers
🏴 1-ounce onion, chopped

🏴 2 ounces sour cream
🏴 tbsp. olive oil

🏴 Salt to taste

Directions:

1. Take a pan and place it over medium heat
2. Add oil and let it heat up
3. Add onions and fry until just browned
4. Add livers and season with salt
5. Cook until livers are half cooked
6. Transfer the mix to a stew pot
7. Add sour cream and cook for 20 min
8. Serve and enjoy!

Nutrition: Calories: 146 Fat: 9g Carbs: 2g Protein: 15g

128.   CHICKEN AND MUSHROOM STEW

Preparation Time: 10 min   **Cooking Time**: 35 min   **Servings**: 4

Ingredients:

🏴 4 chicken breast halves, cut into bite-sized pieces

🏴 pound mushrooms, sliced (5-6 cups)
🏴 bunch spring onion, chopped

🏴 4 tbsp. olive oil
🏴 tsp. thyme
🏴 Salt and pepper as needed

Directions:

1. Take a large deep frying pan and place it over medium-high heat
2. Add oil and let it heat up
3. Add chicken and cook for 4-5 min per side until slightly browned

4. Add spring onions and mushrooms, season with salt and pepper according to your taste

5. Stir. Cover with lid and bring the mix to a boil
6. Lower heat and simmer for 25 mins. Serve!

Nutrition: Calories: 247 Fat: 12g Carbs: 10g Protein: 23g

129. ROASTED CARROT SOUP

Preparation Time: 10 min   **Cooking Time**: 50 min   **Servings**: 4

Ingredients:

- 8 large carrots, washed and peeled
- 6 tbsp. olive oil
- 1-quart broth
- Cayenne pepper to taste
- Salt and pepper to taste

Directions:

1. Preheat your oven to 425 °F
2. Take a baking sheet and add carrots, drizzle olive oil and roast for 30-45 min
3. Put roasted carrots into a blender and add the broth, puree
4. Pour into saucepan and heat soup
5. Season with salt, pepper, and cayenne
6. Drizzle olive oil
7. Serve and enjoy!

Nutrition: Calories: 222 Fat: 18g Net Carbs: 7g Protein: 5g

130. GARLIC AND BUTTER COD

Preparation Time: 5 min   **Cooking Time**: 20 min   **Servings**: 3

Ingredients:

- 3 Cod fillets, 8 ounces each
- ¾ pound baby bock choy halved
- 1/3 cup almond butter, thinly sliced
- 1 1/2 tbsp. garlic, minced
- Salt and pepper to taste

Directions:

1. Preheat your oven to 400 °F
2. Cut 3 sheets of aluminum foil (large enough to fit fillet)
3. Place cod fillet on each sheet and add butter and garlic on top
4. Add bok choy, season with pepper and salt
5. Fold packet and enclose them in pouches
6. Arrange on baking sheet
7. Bake for 20 min
8. Transfer to a cooling rack and let them cool
9. Enjoy!

Nutrition: Calories: 355 Fat: 21g Carbs: 3g Protein: 37g

131. BROCCOLI PLATTER

Preparation Time: 4 min   **Cooking Time**: 14 min   **Servings**: 2

Ingredients:

- 6 ounces of tilapia, frozen
- 1 tbsp. of almond butter
- 1 tbsp. of garlic, minced
- 1 tsp. of lemon pepper seasoning
- 1 cup of broccoli florets, fresh

Directions:

1. Preheat your oven to 350 °F
2. Add fish in aluminum foil packets
3. Arrange the broccoli around fish
4. Sprinkle lemon pepper on top
5. Close the packets and seal
6. Bake for 14 min
7. Take a bowl and add garlic and butter, mix well and keep the mixture on the side
8. Remove the packet from the oven and transfer to a platter
9. Place butter on top of the fish and broccoli, serve and enjoy!

Nutrition: Calories: 362 Fat: 25g Carbs: 2g Protein: 29g

132. ASPARAGUS FRITTATA

Preparation time: 5 mins.   **Cooking time**: 30 mins.   **Servings**: 2

Ingredients:

- 10 medium asparagus spears end trimmed
- 2 tsp. extra-virgin olive oil, divided
- Freshly ground black pepper
- Four large eggs
- ½ tsp. onion powder
- ¼ cup chopped parsley

Directions:

1. Preheat the oven to 450°F.
2. Toss the asparagus with one tsp. of olive oil and season with pepper. Transfer to a baking pan and roast, occasionally stirring, for 20 mins, up until the spears are browned and tender. In a small container, beat the eggs with the onion powder and parsley, season with pepper. Slice the asparagus spears into 1-inch pieces and arrange in a medium skillet. Drizzle with the remaining oil, and shake the pan to distribute.
3. Pour the egg mixture into the skillet, and cook over medium heat. When the egg is well set on the bottom and nearly set on the top, cover it with a plate, invert the pan, so the frittata is on the plate, and then slide it back into the pan with the cooked side up. Remain to cook for about 30 more seconds, until firm.

Nutrition: Calories: 102kcal Total Fat: 8g Saturated Fat: 2g Cholesterol: 104mg Carbs: 4g Fiber: 2g Protein: 6g Phosphorus: 103mg Potassium: 248mg Sodium: 46mg

133. SWEET PANCAKES

Preparation time: 10 mins.   **Cooking time**: 5 mins.   **Servings**: 5

Ingredients:

- 1 cup all-purpose flour
- 1 tbsp. granulated sugar
- Baking powder
- 2 egg whites
- 1 cup almond milk
- 2 tbsp. Olive oil
- 1 tbsp. maple extract

Directions:

1. In a bowl mix the flour, sugar and baking powder. Make a well in the center and place to one side.
2. Mix the egg whites, milk, oil, and maple extract in a separate bowl.
3. Add the egg mixture to the well and gently mix until a batter is formed. Heat skillet over medium heat. Add 1/5 of the batter to the pan and cook 2 minon each side or until the pancake is golden.
4. Repeat with the remaining batter and serve

Nutrition: Calories: 178kcal Fat: 6g Carb: 25g Phosphorus: 116mg Potassium: 126mg Sodium: 297mg Protein: 6g

134. BREAKFAST SMOOTHIE

Preparation time: 15 mins.

Cooking time: 0 mins.

Servings: 2

Ingredients:

- 1 cup frozen blueberries
- ½ cup pineapple chunks
- ½ cup English cucumber
- ½ apple
- ½ cup water

Directions:

1. Put the pineapple, blueberries, cucumber, apple, and water in a blender and blend until thick and smooth.
2. Pour into 2 glasses and serve.

Nutrition: Calories: 87kcal Fat: g Carb: 22g Phosphorus: 28mg Potassium: 192mg Sodium: 3mg Protein: 0.7g

135. POACHED EGGS WITH CILANTRO BUTTER

Preparation time: 5 mins.   **Cooking time**: 10 mins.   **Servings**: 2

Ingredients:

- 2 tbsp. unsalted butter
- 1 tbsp. chopped parsley
- 1 tbsp. chopped cilantro
- 4 large eggs
- Dash vinegar
- Freshly ground black pepper

Directions:

1. In a small pan over low heat, thaw the butter. Add the parsley and cilantro, and cook for about 1 min, stirring constantly. Remove from the heat, and pour it into a small dish.
2. In a small saucepan, bring about 3 inches of water to a simmer. Add the dash of vinegar.
3. Crash one egg into a cup or ramekin. Using a spoon, create a whirlpool in the simmering water, and then pour the egg into the water.

Use the spoon to draw the white together until just starting to set. Repeat with the remaining eggs. Cook for 4 to 7 mins, depending on how to set you like your yolk.

4. With a slotted spoon, remove the eggs.
5. Serve the eggs topped with one tbsp. of the herbed butter and some pepper.

Nutrition: Calories: 261kcal Total Fat: 22g Saturated Fat: 7g Cholesterol: 429mg Carbs: 1g Fiber: 0g Protein: 14g Phosphorus: 226mg Potassium: 173mg Sodium: 164mg

136. EGG AND VEGGIE MUFFINS

Preparation time: 15 mins.   **Cooking time**: 20 mins.   **Servings**: 4

Ingredients:
- Cooking spray
- 4 eggs
- 2 tbsp. unsweetened rice milk
- ½ sweet onion, chopped
- ½ red bell pepper, chopped
- Pinch red pepper flakes
- Pinch ground black pepper
- ¼ cup parsley, diced

Directions:
1. Preheat the oven to 350F.
2. Spray 4 muffin pans with cooking spray. Set aside. Whisk together the milk, eggs, onion, red pepper, red pepper flakes, and black pepper until mixed in a bowl.
3. Pour the egg mixture into prepared muffin pans.
4. Bake until the muffins are puffed and golden, about 18 to 20 mins.
5. Add parsley and Serve.

Nutrition: Calories: 84kcal Fat: 5g Carb: 3g Phosphorus: 110mg Potassium: 117mg Sodium: 75mg Protein: 7g

137. PARSLEY SCALLOPS

Preparation Time: 5 min   **Cooking Time**: 25 min   **Servings**: 4

Ingredients:
- 8 tbsp. almond butter
- 2 garlic cloves, minced
- 16 large sea scallops
- Salt and pepper to taste
- 1 1/2 tbsp. olive oil

Directions:
1. Seasons scallops with salt and pepper
2. Take a skillet and place it over medium heat, add oil and let it heat up Sauté scallops for 2 min per side, repeat until all scallops are cooked
3. Add butter to the skillet and let it melt
4. Stir in garlic and cook for 15 min
5. Return scallops to skillet and stir to coat
6. Serve and enjoy!

Nutrition: Calories: 417 Fat: 31g Net Carbs: 5g Protein: 29g

138. BLACKENED CHICKEN

Preparation Time: 10 min   **Cooking Time**: 10 min   **Servings**: 4

Ingredients:
- 1/2 tsp. paprika
- 1/8 tsp. salt
- 1/4 tsp. cayenne pepper
- 1/4 tsp. ground cumin
- 1/4 tsp. dried thyme
- 1/8 tsp. ground white pepper
- 1/8 tsp. onion powder
- 2 chicken breasts, boneless and skinless

Directions:
1. Preheat your oven to 350 °F
2. Grease baking sheet
3. Take a cast-iron skillet and place it over high heat Add oil and heat it up for 5 min until smoking hot
4. Take a small bowl and mix salt, paprika, cumin, white pepper, cayenne, thyme, onion powder
5. Oil the chicken breast on both sides and coat the breast with the spice mix
6. Transfer to your hot pan and cook for 1 min per side
7. Transfer to your prepared baking sheet and bake for 5 min
8. Serve and enjoy!

Nutrition: Calories: 136 Fat: 3g Carbs: 1g Protein: 24g

139. SPICY PAPRIKA LAMB CHOPS

Preparation Time: 10 min **Cooking Time**: 15 min **Servings**: 4

Ingredients:

- 2 lamb racks, cut into chops
- Salt and pepper to taste
- 3 tbsp. paprika
- ¾ cup cumin powder
- 1 tsp. chili powder

Directions:

1. Take a bowl and add the paprika, cumin, chili, salt, pepper, and stir. Add lamb chops and rub the mixture
2. Heat grill over medium-temperature and add lamb chops, cook for 5 min
3. Flip and cook for 5 min more, flip again
4. Cook for 2 mins, flip and cook for 2 min more
5. Serve and enjoy!

Nutrition: Calories: 200 Fat: 5g Carbs: 4g Protein: 8g

140. MUSHROOM AND OLIVE STEAK

Preparation Time: 10 min **Cooking Time**: 14 min **Servings**: 4

Ingredients:

- 1 pound boneless beef sirloin steak, ¾ inch thick, cut into 4 pieces
- 1 large red onion, chopped
- 1 cup mushrooms
- 4 garlic cloves, thinly sliced
- 4 tbsp. olive oil
- 1 cup parsley leaves, finely cut

Directions:

1. Take a large-sized skillet and place it over medium-high heat. Add oil and let it heat up
2. Add beef and cook until both sides are browned, remove beef and drain fat
3. Add the rest of the oil to skillet and heat it up
4. Add onions, garlic and cook for 2-3 min. Stir well.
5. Return beef to skillet and lower heat to medium
6. Cook for 3-4 min(covered)
7. Stir in parsley
8. Serve and enjoy!

Nutrition: Calories: 386 Fat: 30g Carbs: 11g Protein: 21g

141. PARSLEY AND CHICKEN BREAST

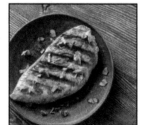

Preparation Time: 10 min
Cooking Time: 40 min
Servings: 4
Ingredients:

- 1 tbsp. dry parsley
- 1 tbsp. dry basil
- 4 chicken breast halves, boneless and skinless
- 1/2 tsp. salt
- 1/2 tsp. red pepper flakes, crushed

Directions:

1. Preheat your oven to 350 °F
2. Take a 9x13 inch baking dish and grease it with cooking spray. Sprinkle 1 tbsp. of parsley, 1 tsp. of basil and spread the mixture over your baking dish. Arrange the chicken breast halves over the dish and sprinkle garlic slices on top
3. Take a small bowl and add 1 tsp. parsley, 1 tsp. of basil, salt, basil, red pepper and mix well. Pour the mixture over the chicken breast
4. Bake for 25 min
5. Remove the cover and bake for 15 min more
6. Serve and enjoy!

Nutrition: Calories: 150 Fat: 4g Carbs: 4g Protein: 25g

CHAPTER 8. FISH AND SEAFOOD

142. CURRIED FISH CAKES

Preparation Time: 10 min.　　　**Cooking Time:** 18 min.　　　**Servings**: 4

Ingredients:

- ¾ pound Atlantic cod, cubed
- 1 apple, peeled and cubed
- 1 tbsp. yellow curry paste
- 2 tbsp. cornstarch
- 1 tbsp. peeled grated ginger root
- 1 large egg
- 1 tbsp. freshly squeezed lemon juice
- 1/8 tsp. freshly ground black pepper
- ½ cup crushed puffed rice cereal
- 1 tbsp. olive oil

Directions:

1. Put the cod, apple, curry, cornstarch, ginger, egg, lemon juice, and pepper in a blender or food processor and process until finely chopped. Avoid over-processing, or the mixture will become mushy. Place the rice cereal on a shallow plate.
2. Form the mixture into 8 patties.
3. Dredge the patties in the rice cereal to coat.
4. Cook patties for 3 to 5 min. per side, turning once until a meat thermometer registers 160°F. Serve.

Nutrition - Per Serving: Per Serving: Calories: 188; Total fat: 6g; Saturated fat: 1g; Sodium: 150mg; Potassium: 292mg; Phosphorus: 150mg; Carbs: 12g; Fiber: 1g; Protein: 21g; Sugar: 5g

143. BAKED SOLE WITH CARAMELIZED ONION

Preparation Time: 10 min.　　　**Cooking Time:** 20 min.　　　**Servings**: 4

Ingredients:

- 1 cup finely chopped onion
- ½ cup low-sodium vegetable broth
- 1 yellow summer squash, sliced
- 2 cups frozen broccoli florets
- 4 (3-ounce) fillets of sole
- Pinch salt
- 2 tbsp. olive oil
- Pinch baking soda
- 2 tsp. avocado oil
- 1 tsp. dried basil leaves

Directions:

1. Preheat the oven to 425°F.
2. Add the onions. Cook for 1 min.; then, stirring constantly, cook for another 4 min.
3. Remove the onions from the heat.
4. Pour the broth into a baking sheet with a lip and arrange the squash and broccoli on the sheet in a single layer. Top the vegetables with the fish. Sprinkle the fish with the salt and drizzle everything with the olive oil.
5. Bake the fish and the vegetables for 10 min.
6. While the fish is baking, return the skillet with the onions to medium-high heat and stir in a pinch of baking soda. Stir in the avocado oil and cook for 5 min., stirring frequently, until the onions are dark brown.
7. Transfer the onions to a plate.
8. Top the fish evenly with the onions. Sprinkle with the basil. Return the fish to the oven, after this bake it 8 to 10 min. Serve the fish on the vegetables.

Nutrition - Per Serving: Per Serving: Calories: 202; Total fat: 11g; Saturated fat: 3g; Sodium: 320mg; Potassium: 537; Phosphorus: 331mg; Carbs: 10g; Fiber: 3g; Protein: 16g; Sugar: 4g

144.   THAI TUNA WRAPS

Preparation Time: 10 min.   **Cooking Time:** 0 min.   **Servings**: 4

Ingredients:

- ¼ cup unsalted peanut butter
- 2 tbsp. freshly squeezed lemon juice
- 1 tsp. low-sodium soy sauce
- ½ tsp. ground ginger
- 1/8 tsp. cayenne pepper
- 1 (6-ounce) can no-salt-added or low-sodium chunk light tuna, drained
- 1 cup shredded red cabbage
- 2 scallions, white and green parts, chopped
- 1 cup grated carrots
- 8 butter lettuce leaves

Directions:

1. In a medium bowl, stir together the peanut butter, lemon juice, soy sauce, ginger, and cayenne pepper until well combined.
2. Stir in the tuna, cabbage, scallions, and carrots.
3. Divide the tuna filling evenly between the butter lettuce leaves and serve.

Nutrition - Per Serving: Per Serving: Calories: 175; Total fat; 10g; Saturated fat: 1g; Sodium: 98mg; Potassium: 421mg; Phosphorus: 153mg; Carbs: 8g; Fiber: 2g; Protein: 17g; Sugar: 4g

145.   GRILLED FISH AND VEGETABLE PACKETS

Preparation Time: 15 min.   **Cooking Time:** 12 min.   **Servings**: 4

Ingredients:

- 1 (8-ounce) package sliced mushrooms
- 1 leek, white and green parts, chopped
- 1 cup frozen corn
- 4 (4-ounce) Atlantic cod fillets
- Juice of 1 lemon
- 3 tbsp. olive oil

Directions:

1. Prepare and preheat the grill to medium coals and set a grill 6 inches from the coals.
2. Tear off four 30-inch long strips of heavy-duty aluminum foil. Arrange the mushrooms, leek, and corn in the center of each piece of foil and top with the fish. Drizzle the packet contents evenly with the lemon juice and olive oil.
3. Bring the longer length sides of the foil together at the top and, holding the edges together, fold them over twice and then fold in the width sides to form a sealed packet with room for the steam.
4. Put the packets on the grill and grill for 10 to 12 min. until the vegetables are tender-crisp and the fish flakes when tested with a fork. Be careful opening the packets because the escaping steam can be scalding.

Nutrition - Per Serving: Per Serving: Calories: 267; Total fat: 12g; Saturated fat: 2g; Sodium: 97mg; Potassium: 582mg; Phosphorus: 238mg; Carbs: 13g; Fiber: 2g; Protein: 29g; Sugar: 3g

146.   WHITE FISH SOUP

Preparation Time: 15 min.   **Cooking Time:** 20 min.   **Servings**:

Ingredients:

- 2 tbsp. olive oil
- 1 onion, fincly diced
- 1 green bell pepper, chopped
- 1 rib celery, thinly sliced
- 3 cups chicken broth, or more to taste
- 1/4 cup chopped fresh parsley
- 1 1/2 pounds cod, cut into 3/4-inch cubes
- Pepper to taste
- 1 dash red pepper flakes

Directions:

1. Heat oil in a soup pot over medium heat.
2. Add onion, bell pepper, and celery and cook until wilted, about 5 min.
3. Add broth and then bring to a simmer, about 5 min. Cook 15 to 20 min.

4. Add cod, parsley, and red pepper flakes and simmer until fish flakes easily with a fork, 8 to 10 min. more. Season with black pepper.

Nutrition - Per Serving: Calories: 117, Total Fat 7.2g, Saturated Fat 1.4g, Cholesterol 18mg, Sodium 37mg, Total Carbs 5.4g, Dietary Fiber 1.3g, Total Sugars 2.8g, Protein 8.1g, Calcium 23mg, Iron 1mg, Potassium 122mg, Phosphorus 111 mg

147. LEMON BUTTER SALMON

Preparation Time: 15 min.   **Cooking Time:** 15 min.   **Servings**: 6

Ingredients:
- 1 tbsp. butter
- 2 tbsp. olive oil
- 1 tbsp. Dijon mustard
- 1 tbsp. lemon juice
- 2 cloves garlic, crushed
- 1 tsp. dried dill
- 1 tsp. dried basil leaves
- 1 tbsp. capers
- 24-ounce salmon filet

Directions:
1. Put all of the ingredients except the salmon in a saucepan over medium heat.
2. Bring to a boil and then simmer for 5 min.
3. Preheat your grill.
4. Create a packet using foil.
5. Place the sauce and salmon inside.
6. Seal the packet.
7. Grill for 12 min.

Nutrition - Per Serving: Calories: 292 Protein 22 g Carbs 2 g Fat 22 g Cholesterol 68 mg Sodium 190 mg Potassium 439 mg Phosphorus 280 mg Calcium 21 mg

148. CRAB CAKE

Preparation Time: 15 min.   **Cooking Time:** 9 min.   **Servings**: 6

Ingredients:
- 1/4 cup onion, chopped
- 1/4 cup bell pepper, chopped
- 1 egg, beaten
- 6 low-sodium crackers, crushed
- 1/4 cup low-fat mayonnaise
- 1-pound crab meat
- 1 tbsp. dry mustard
- Pepper to taste
- 2 tbsp. lemon juice
- 1 tbsp. fresh parsley
- 1 tbsp. garlic powder
- 3 tbsp. olive oil

Directions:
1. Mix all the ingredients except the oil.
2. Form 6 patties from the mixture.
3. Pour the oil into a pan in a medium heat.
4. Cook the crab cakes for 5 min.
5. Flip and cook for another 4 min.

Nutrition - Per Serving: Calories: 189 Protein 13 g Carbs 5 g Fat 14 g Cholesterol 111 mg Sodium 342 mg Potassium 317 mg Phosphorus 185 mg Calcium 52 mg Fiber 0.5 g

149. BAKED FISH IN CREAM SAUCE

Preparation Time: 10 min.   **Cooking Time:** 40 min.   **Servings**: 4

Ingredients:

- 1-pound haddock
- 1/2 cup all-purpose flour
- 2 tbsp. butter (unsalted)
- 1/4 tsp. pepper
- 2 cups fat-free nondairy creamer
- 1/4 cup water

Directions:

1. Preheat your oven to 350 F.
2. Spray baking pan with oil.
3. Sprinkle with a little flour.
4. Arrange fish on the pan
5. Season with pepper.
6. Sprinkle remaining flour on the fish.
7. Spread creamer on both sides of the fish.
8. Bake for 40 min. or until golden.
9. Spread cream sauce on top of the fish before serving.

Nutrition - Per Serving: Calories: 383 Protein 24 g Carbs 46 g Fat 11 g Cholesterol 79 mg Sodium 253 mg Potassium 400 mg Phosphorus 266 mg Calcium 46 mg Fiber 0.4 g

150.   SHRIMP & BROCCOLI

Preparation Time: 10 min.   **Cooking Time:** 5 min.   **Servings**: 4

Ingredients:

- 1 tbsp. olive oil
- 1 clove garlic, minced
- 1-pound shrimp
- 1/4 cup red bell pepper
- 1 cup broccoli florets, steamed
- 10-ounce cream cheese
- 1/2 tsp. garlic powder
- 1/4 cup lemon juice
- 3/4 tsp. ground peppercorns
- 1/4 cup half and half creamer

Directions:

1. Pour the oil and cook garlic for 30 seconds.
2. Add shrimp and cook for 2 min.
3. Add the rest of the ingredients.
4. Mix well.
5. Cook for 2 min.

Nutrition - Per Serving: Calories: 469 Protein 28 g Carbs 28 g Fat 28 g Cholesterol 213 mg Sodium 374 mg Potassium 469 mg Phosphorus 335 mg Calcium 157 mg Fiber 2.6 g

151.   SHRIMP IN GARLIC SAUCE

Preparation Time: 10 min.   **Cooking Time:** 6 min.   **Servings**: 4

Ingredients:

- 3 tbsp. butter (unsalted)
- 1/4 cup onion, minced
- 3 cloves garlic, minced
- 1-pound shrimp, shelled and deveined
- 1/2 cup half and half creamer
- 1/4 cup white wine
- 2 tbsp. fresh basil
- Black pepper to taste

Directions:

1. Add butter to a pan over medium low heat.
2. Let it melt.
3. Add the onion and garlic. Cook for it 1-2 min. Add the shrimp and cook for 2 min. Transfer shrimp on a serving platter and set aside.
4. Add the rest of the ingredients.

5. Simmer for 3 min.

6. Pour sauce over the shrimp and serve.

Nutrition - Per Serving: Calories: 482 Protein 33 g Carbs 46 g Fat 11 g Cholesterol 230 mg Sodium 213 mg Potassium 514 mg Phosphorus 398 mg Calcium 133 mg Fiber 2.0 g

152. FISH TACO

Preparation Time: 40 min.   **Cooking Time:** 10 min.   **Servings**: 6

Ingredients:

- 1 tbsp. lime juice
- 1 tbsp. olive oil
- 1 clove garlic, minced
- 1-pound cod fillets
- 1/2 tsp. ground cumin
- 1/4 tsp. black pepper
- 1/2 tsp. chili powder
- 1/4 cup sour cream
- 1/2 cup mayonnaise
- 2 tbsp. nondairy milk
- 1 cup cabbage, shredded
- 1/2 cup onion, chopped
- 1/2 bunch cilantro, chopped
- 12 corn tortillas

Directions:

1. Drizzle lemon juice over the fish fillet.
2. And then coat it with olive oil and then season with garlic, cumin, pepper and chili powder.
3. Let it sit for 30 min.
4. Broil fish for 10 min., flipping halfway through.
5. Flake the fish using a fork.
6. In a bowl, mix sour cream, milk and mayo.
7. Assemble tacos by filling each tortilla with mayo mixture, cabbage, onion, cilantro and fish flakes.

Nutrition - Per Serving: Calories: 366 Protein 18 g Carbs 31 g Fat 19 g Cholesterol 40 mg Sodium 194 mg Potassium 507 mg Phosphorus 327 mg Calcium 138 mg Fiber 4.3 g

153. BAKED TROUT

Preparation Time: 5 min.   **Cooking Time:** 10 min.   **Servings**: 8

Ingredients:

- 2-pound trout fillet
- 1 tbsp. oil
- 1 tsp. salt-free lemon pepper
- 1/2 tsp. paprika

Directions:

1. Preheat your oven to 350 F.
2. Coat fillet with oil.
3. Place fish on a baking pan.
4. Season with lemon pepper and paprika.
5. Bake for 10 min.

Nutrition - Per Serving: Calories: 161 Protein 21 g Carbs 0 g Fat 8 g Cholesterol 58 mg Sodium 109 mg Potassium 385 mg Phosphorus 227 mg Calcium 75 mg Fiber 0.1 g

154. FISH WITH MUSHROOMS

Preparation Time: 5 min.   **Cooking Time:** 16 min.   **Servings**: 4

Ingredients:

- 1-pound cod fillet
- 2 tbsp. butter

Renal Diet Cookbook

- ¼ cup white onion, chopped
- 1 cup fresh mushrooms
- 1 tsp. dried thyme

Directions:

1. Put the fish in a baking pan.
2. Preheat your oven to 450 F.
3. Melt the butter and cook onion and mushroom for 1 min.
4. Spread mushroom mixture on top of the fish.
5. Season with thyme.
6. Bake in the oven for 15 min.

Nutrition - Per Serving: Calories: 156 Protein 21 g Carbs 3 g Fat 7 g Cholesterol 49 mg Sodium 110 mg Potassium 561 mg Phosphorus 225 mg Calcium 30 mg Fiber 0.5 g

155.   SALMON WITH SPICY HONEY

Preparation Time: 15 Min.   **Cooking Time:** 8 min.   **Servings**: 2

Ingredients:

- 16-ounce salmon fillet
- 3 tbsp. honey
- 3/4 tsp. lemon peel
- 3 bowls arugula salad
- 1/2 tsp. black pepper
- 1/2 tsp. garlic powder
- 2 tsp. olive oil
- 1 tsp. hot water

Directions:

1. Prepare a small bowl with some hot water and put in honey, grated lemon peel, ground pepper, and garlic powder. Spread the mixture over salmon fillets. Warm some olive oil at a medium heat and add spiced salmon fillet and cook for 4 min.
2. Turn the fillets on one side then on the other side.
3. Continue to cook for other 4 min. at a reduced heat and try to check when the salmon fillets flake easily.
4. Put some arugula on each plate and add the salmon fillets on top, adding some aromatic herbs or some dill. Serve and enjoy!

Nutrition - Per Serving: Calories: 320 Protein: 23 g Sodium: 65 mg Potassium: 450 mg Phosphorus: 250 mg

156.   SALMON WITH MAPLE GLAZE

Preparation Time: 15 min.   **Cooking Time:** 2 hs   **Servings**: 4

Ingredients:

- 1-pound salmon fillets
- 1 tbsp. green onion, chopped
- 1 tbsp. low sodium soy sauce
- 2 garlic cloves, pressed
- 2 tbsp. fresh cilantro
- 3 tbsp. lemon juice (or juice of 1 lemon)
- 3 tbsp. maple syrup

Directions:

1. Combine all ingredients except for salmon.
2. Put salmon on platter and then pour marinade over fillets. Let it marinate 2 hs or more.
3. Preheat broiler.
4. Remove salmon from marinade.
5. Place salmon on bottom rack and broil for 10 min. Do not turn over.
6. Serve hot/cold with a wedge of lemon.

Nutrition - Per Serving: Calories: per Serving: 220; Carbs: 12g; protein: 24g; fats: 8g; phosphorus: 374mg; potassium: 440mg; sodium: 621mg

157.   STEAMED SPICY TILAPIA FILLET

Preparation Time: 10 min.   **Cooking Time:** 25 min.   **Servings**: 4

Ingredients:

- 4 fillets of tilapia
- 1 tsp. hot pepper sauce
- 1 large sprig thyme
- 1 tbsp. Ketchup
- 1 tbsp. lime juice

- 1 cup hot water
- 1/2 cup onion, sliced
- 1/4 tsp. black pepper
- 3/4 cup red and green peppers, sliced

Directions:

1. A large shallow dish that fits your steamer, mix well hot pepper sauce, thyme, ketchup, lemon juice, and black pepper. Mix thoroughly. Add tilapia fillets and spoon over sauce.
2. Mix in remaining ingredients except for water. Mix well in sauce. Cover top of dish with foil.
3. Add the hot water in the steamer. Place dish on steamer rack. Cover pot and steam fish and veggies for 20 min. Let it stand for 5-6 min. before serving.

Nutrition - Per Serving: Calories: per Serving: 131; Carbs: 5g; protein: 24g; fats: 3g; phosphorus: 212mg; potassium: 457mg; sodium: 102mg

158. DIJON MUSTARD AND LIME MARINATED SHRIMP

Preparation Time: 20 min.   **Cooking Time:** 80 min.   **Servings**: 8

Ingredients:

- 1-pound uncooked shrimp, peeled and deveined
- 1 bay leaf
- 3 whole cloves
- ½ cup rice vinegar
- 1 cup water

- ½ tsp. hot sauce
- 2 tbsp. capers
- 2 tbsp. Dijon mustard
- ½ cup fresh lime juice, plus lime zest as garnish
- 1 medium red onion, chopped

Directions:

1. Mix hot sauce, mustard, capers, lime juice and onion in a shallow baking dish and set aside.
2. Bring it to a boil in a large saucepan bay leaf, cloves, vinegar and water.
3. Once boiling, add shrimps and cook for a min. while stirring continuously.
4. Drain shrimps and pour shrimps into onion mixture.
5. For an h, refrigerate while covered the shrimps.
6. Then serve shrimps cold and garnished with lime zest.

Nutrition - Per Serving: Calories: per Serving: 123; Carbs: 3g; protein: 12g; fats: 1g; phosphorus: 119mg; potassium: 87mg; sodium: 568mg

159. BAKED COD CRUSTED WITH HERBS

Preparation Time: 15 min.   **Cooking Time:** 10 min.   **Servings**: 4

Ingredients:

- ¼ cup honey
- ½ cup panko
- ½ tsp. pepper
- 1 tbsp. extra-virgin olive oil
- 1 tbsp. lemon juice

- 1 tsp. dried basil
- 1 tsp. dried parsley
- 1 tsp. rosemary
- 4 pieces of 4-ounce cod fillets

Directions:

1. With olive oil, grease a 9 x 13-inch baking pan and preheat oven to 375oF.
2. In a zip top bag mix panko, rosemary, pepper, parsley and basil.
3. Evenly spread cod fillets in prepped dish and drizzle with lemon juice.
4. Then brush the fillets with honey on all sides. Discard remaining honey if any.
5. Then evenly divide the panko mixture on top of cod fillets.
6. Pop in the oven and bake for ten min. or until fish is cooked. Serve and enjoy.

Nutrition - Per Serving: Calories: per Serving: 113; Carbs: 21g; protein: 5g; fats: 2g; phosphorus: 89mg; potassium: 115mg; sodium: 139mg

160. DILL RELISH ON WHITE SEA BASS

Preparation Time: 15 min.   **Cooking Time:** 60 min.   **Servings**: 4

Ingredients:

- 1 lemon, quartered
- 4 pieces of 4-ounce white sea bass fillets
- 1 tsp. lemon juice
- 1 tsp. Dijon mustard
- 1 ½ tsp.. chopped fresh dill
- 1 tsp. pickled baby capers, drained
- 1 ½ tbsp. chopped white onion

Directions:

1. Preheat oven to 375oF. Mix lemon juice, mustard, dill, capers and onions in a small bowl. Prepare four aluminum foil squares and place 1 fillet per foil. Squeeze a lemon wedge per fish.
2. Evenly divide into 4 the dill spread and drizzle over fillet.
3. Close the foil over the fish securely and pop in the oven. Bake for 9 to 12 min. or until fish is cooked through.
4. Remove from foil and transfer to a serving platter, serve and enjoy.

Nutrition - Per Serving: Calories: per Serving: 71; Carbs: 11g; protein: 7g; fats: 1g; phosphorus: 91mg; potassium: 237mg; sodium: 94mg

161. TILAPIA WITH LEMON GARLIC SAUCE

Preparation Time: 15 min.   **Cooking Time:** 30 min.   **Servings**: 4

Ingredients:

- Pepper
- 1 tsp. dried parsley flakes
- 1 clove garlic (finely chopped)
- 1 tbsp. butter (melted)
- 3 tbsp. fresh lemon juice
- 4 tilapia fillets

Directions:

1. First, spray baking dish with non-stick cooking spray then preheat oven at 375 Fahrenheit (190oC).
2. In cool water, rinse tilapia fillets and using paper towels pat dry the fillets.
3. Place tilapia fillets in the baking dish, pour butter and lemon juice and top off with pepper, parsley and garlic.
4. Bake tilapia in the preheated oven for 30 min. and wait until fish is white.
5. Enjoy!

Nutrition - Per Serving: Calories: per Serving: 168; Carbs: 4g; protein: 24g; fats: 5g; phosphorus: 207mg; potassium: 431mg; sodium: 85mg

162. SPINACH WITH TUSCAN WHITE BEANS AND SHRIMPS

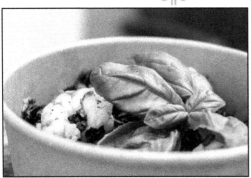

Preparation Time: 5 min.
Cooking Time: 15 min.
Servings: 4
Nutrition - Per Serving:
Calories: 343
Carbs: 21g
Protein: 22g
Fats: 11g
Phosphorus: 400mg
Potassium: 599mg
Sodium: 766mg

Ingredients:
- 1 ½ ounces crumbled reduce-fat feta cheese
- 5 cups baby spinach
- 15 ounces can no salt added cannellini beans (rinsed and drained)
- ½ cup low sodium, fat-free chicken broth
- 2 tbsp. balsamic vinegar
- 2 tsp. chopped fresh sage
- 4 cloves garlic (minced)
- 1 medium onion (chopped)
- 1-pound large shrimp (peeled and deveined)
- 2 tbsp. olive oil

Directions:
1. Heat 1 tsp. oil. Heat it over medium-high.
2. Then for about 2 to 3 min., cook the shrimps using the heated skillet then place them on a plate. Heat on the same skillet the sage, garlic, and onions then cook for about 4 min. Add and stir in vinegar for 30 seconds.
3. For about 2 min., add chicken broth. Then, add spinach and beans and cook for an additional 2 to 3 min.
4. Remove skillet then add and stir in cooked shrimps topped with feta cheese.
5. Serve and divide into 4 bowls. Enjoy!

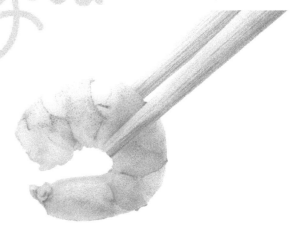

163. SALMON STUFFED PASTA

Preparation Time: 20 min. **Cooking Time:** 35 min. **Servings**: 24

Ingredients:

- 24 jumbo pasta shells, boiled
- 1 cup coffee creamer

FILLING:

- 2 eggs, beaten
- 2 cups creamed cottage cheese

- ¼ cup chopped onion
- 1 red bell pepper, diced
- 2 tsp. dried parsley
- ½ tsp. lemon peel
- 1 can salmon, drained

DILL SAUCE:

- 1 ½ tsp. butter
- 1 ½ tsp. flour
- 1/8 tsp. pepper
- 1 tbsp. lemon juice
- 1 ½ cup coffee creamer
- 2 tsp. dried dill weed

Directions:

1. Beat the cream cheese with the egg and all the other filling ingredients in a bowl.
2. Divide the filling in the pasta shells and place the shells in a 9x13 baking dish. Pour the coffee creamer around the stuffed shells then cover with a foil.
3. Bake the shells for 30 min. at 350 F. Meanwhile, whisk all the ingredients for dill sauce in a saucepan.
4. Stir for 5 min. until it thickens. Pour this sauce over the baked pasta shells.
5. Serve warm.

Nutrition - Per Serving: Calories: 268; Fat: 4.8g; Sodium 86mg; Protein 11.5g; Calcium 27mg; Phosphorous 314mg; Potassium 181mg

164. BAGEL WITH SALMON AND EGG

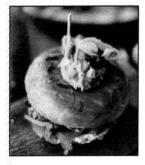

Preparation Time: 15 min.
Cooking Time: 10 min.
Servings: 1
Nutrition - Per Serving:

Protein: 19 g
Fat: 14 g
Carbs: 29 g
Cholesterol: 218 mg
Potassium: 338 mg

Sodium: 378 mg
Phosphorus: 270 mg
Fiber: 2.6 g
Calcium: 77 mg

Ingredients:

- ½ Bagel
- 1 tbsp. Cream cheese
- 1 tbsp. Scallions
- ½ tsp. Fresh dill

- 2 Fresh basil leaves
- 1 slice Tomato
- 4 pieces Arugula
- 1 large Egg

- 1-ounce Cooked salmon

Directions:

1. Start by slicing the bagel through the center horizontally. Take one half of the bagel and toast it in an oven or a toaster.
2. Finely chop the dill, basil leaves, and scallions. Set aside. Add in the cream cheese. Toss in the chopped dill, basil, and scallions. Mix well to combine. Take the toasted bagel and spread the herbs and cream cheese mixture evenly over it.
3. Place the tomato slice and arugula on top. Set aside. Take a small mixing bowl and then beat the egg.
   Take a non-stick saucepan and grease it using cooking spray. Stir after pouring the beaten egg into the pan and. Cook for about 1 min. over medium heat. Keep stirring to make a perfect scrambled egg.
4. Take the cooked salmon and place it in the same pan as the egg. This will help you heat the

salmon and cook the egg at the same time.
Place the scrambled egg over the tomato slice
and top it with the salmon

165.   HERBED VEGETABLE TROUT

Preparation Time: 15 min.   **Cooking Time:** 15 min.   **Servings**: 4

Ingredients:

- 14 oz. trout fillets
- 1/2 tsp. herb seasoning blend
- 1 lemon, sliced
- 2 green onions, sliced
- 1 stalk celery, chopped
- 1 medium carrot, julienne

Directions:

1. Prepare and preheat a charcoal grill over moderate heat. Place the trout fillets over a large piece of foil and drizzle herb seasoning on top.
2. Spread the lemon slices, carrots, celery, and green onions over the fish.
3. Cover the fish with foil and pack it.
4. Place the packed fish in the grill and cook for 15 min.
5. Once done, remove the foil from the fish.
6. Serve.

Nutrition - Per Serving: Calories: 202; Fat 8.5g; Sodium 82mg; Calcium 70mg ; Phosphorous 287mg; Potassium 560mg

166.   CITRUS GLAZED SALMON

Preparation Time: 20 min.   **Cooking Time:** 17 min.   **Servings**: 4

Ingredients:

- 2 garlic cloves, crushed
- 1/2 tbsp. lemon juice
- 2 tbsp. olive oil
- 1 tbsp. butter
- 1 tbsp. Dijon mustard
- 2 dashes cayenne pepper
- 1 tsp. dried basil leaves
- 1 tsp. dried dill
- 24 oz. salmon filet

Directions:

1. Place a 1-quart saucepan over moderate heat and add the oil, butter, garlic, lemon juice, mustard, cayenne pepper, dill, and basil to the pan. Stir this mixture for 5 min. after it has boiled. Prepare and preheat a charcoal grill over moderate heat.
2. Place the fish on a foil sheet and fold the edges to make a foil tray. Pour the prepared sauce over the fish.
3. Place the fish in the foil in the preheated grill and cook for 12 min.
4. Slice and serve.

Nutrition - Per Serving: Calories: 401; Fat 20.5g; Cholesterol 144mg; Sodium 256mg; Carbs 0.5g; Calcium 549mg; Phosphorous 214mg; Potassium 446mg

167.   BROILED SALMON FILLETS

Preparation Time: 10 min.   **Cooking Time:** 13 min.   **Servings**: 4

Ingredients:

- 1 tbsp. ginger root, grated
- 1 clove garlic, minced
- ¼ cup maple syrup
- 1 tbsp. hot pepper sauce
- 4 salmon fillets, skinless

Directions:

1. Grease a pan with cooking spray and place it over moderate heat. Add the ginger and garlic and sauté for 3 min. then transfer to a bowl.
2. Add the hot pepper sauce and maple syrup to the ginger-garlic. Mix well and keep this mixture aside.
3. Place the salmon fillet in a suitable baking tray, greased with cooking oil. Brush the maple sauce over the fillets liberally
4. Broil them for 10 min. at the oven at broiler settings. Serve warm.

Nutrition - Per Serving: Calories: 289; Fat 11.1g; Sodium 80mg; Carbs 13.6g; Calcium 78mg; Phosphorous 230mg; Potassium 331mg

168. BROILED SHRIMP

Preparation Time: 10 min.   **Cooking Time:** 5 min.   **Servings**: 8

Ingredients:

- 1 lb. shrimp in shell
- 1/2 cup unsalted butter, melted
- 2 tsp. lemon juice
- 2 tbsp. chopped onion
- 1 clove garlic, minced
- 1/8 tsp. pepper

Directions:

1. Toss the shrimp with the butter, lemon juice, onion, garlic, and pepper in a bowl.
2. Spread the seasoned shrimp in a baking tray.
3. Broil for 5 min. in an oven on broiler setting.
4. Serve warm.

Nutrition - Per Serving: Calories: 164; Fat 12.8g; Sodium 242mg; Carbs 0.6g; Calcium 45mg; Phosphorous 215mg; Potassium 228mg

169. GRILLED LEMONY COD

Preparation Time: 10 min.   **Cooking Time:** 10 min.   **Servings**: 4

Ingredients:

- 1 lb. cod fillets
- 1 tsp. salt-free lemon pepper seasoning
- 1/4 cup lemon juice

Directions:

1. Rub the cod fillets with lemon pepper seasoning and lemon juice.
2. Grease a baking tray with cooking spray and place the salmon in the baking tray.
3. Bake the fish for 10 min. at 350 F in a preheated oven.
4. Serve warm.

Nutrition - Per Serving: Calories: 155; Fat 7.1g; Cholesterol 50mg; Sodium 53mg; Protein 22.2g; Calcium 43mg Phosphorous 237mg; Potassium 461mg

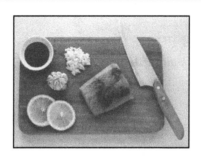

CHAPTER 9. VEGETABLE RECIPES

170.   SPICY MUSHROOM STIR-FRY

Preparation Time: 10 min.   **Cooking Time:** 10 min.   **Servings**: 4

Ingredients:

- 1 cup low-sodium vegetable broth
- 2 tbsp. cornstarch
- 1 tsp. low-sodium soy sauce
- 1/2 tsp. ground ginger
- 1/8 tsp. cayenne pepper
- 2 tbsp. olive oil
- 2 (8-ounce) packages sliced button mushrooms
- 1 red bell pepper, chopped
- 1 jalapeño pepper, minced
- 3 cups brown rice that has been cooked in unsalted water
- 2 tbsp. sesame oil

Directions:

1. In a small bowl, whisk together the broth, cornstarch, soy sauce, ginger, and cayenne pepper and set aside.
2. Heat the olive oil in a wok or heavy skillet over high heat.
3. Add the mushrooms and peppers and stir-fry for 3 to 5 min. or until the vegetables are tender-crisp.
4. Stir the broth mixture and add it to the wok; stir-fry for 3 to 5 min. longer or until the vegetables are tender and the sauce has thickened.
5. Serve the stir-fry over the hot cooked brown rice and drizzle with the sesame oil.

Nutrition - Per Serving: Calories: 36; Fat: 16g; Carbs: 49g; Protein: 8g; Sodium: 95mg; Phosphorus: 267mg; Potassium: 582mg

171.   CURRIED VEGGIES AND RICE

Preparation Time: 12 min.   **Cooking Time:** 18 min.   **Servings**: 4

Ingredients:

- 1/4 cup olive oil
- 1 cup long-grain white basmati rice
- 4 garlic cloves, minced
- 1/2 tsp. curry powder
- 1/2 cup sliced shiitake mushrooms
- 1 red bell pepper, chopped
- 1 cup frozen, shelled edamame
- 2 cups low-sodium vegetable broth
- 1/8 tsp. freshly ground black pepper

Directions:

1. Heat the olive oil on medium heat.
2. Add the rice, garlic, curry powder, mushrooms, bell pepper, and edamame; cook, stirring, for 2 min.
3. Add the broth and black pepper and bring to a boil. Reduce the heat to low, partially cover the pot, and simmer for 15 to 18 min. or until the rice is tender. Stir and serve.

Nutrition - Per Serving: Calories: 347; Fat: 16g; Carbs: 44g; Protein: 8g; Sodium: 114mg; Phosphorus: 131mg; Potassium: 334mg

172.   SPICY VEGGIE PANCAKES

Preparation Time: 10 min.   **Cooking Time:** 10 min.   **Servings**: 4

Ingredients:

- 3 tbsp. olive oil, divided
- 2 small onions, finely chopped
- 1 jalapeño pepper, minced
- 3/4 cup carrot, grated
- 3/4 cup cabbage, finely chopped
- 11/2 cups quick-cooking oats

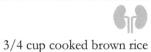
- 3/4 cup cooked brown rice
- 3/4 cup of water
- ½ cup whole-wheat flour
- 1 large egg
- 1 large egg white
- 1 tsp. baking soda
- 1/4 tsp. cayenne pepper

Directions:

1. In a skillet, heat 2 tsp. oil over medium heat. Sauté the onion, jalapeño, carrot, and cabbage for 4 min.
2. While the veggies are cooking, combine the oats, rice, water, flour, egg, egg white, baking soda, and cayenne pepper in a medium bowl until well mixed.
3. Add the cooked vegetables to the mixture and stir to combine.
4. Heat the remaining oil in a large skillet over medium heat.
5. Drop the mixture into the skillet, about 1/3 cup per pancake. Cook for 4 min., or until bubbles form on the pancakes' surface and the edges look cooked, then carefully flip them over.
6. Repeat with the remaining mixture and serve.

Nutrition - Per Serving: Calories: 323; Fat: 11g; Carbs: 48g; Protein: 10g; Sodium: 366mg; Potassium: 381mg; Phosphorus: 263mg

---

173.   EGG AND VEGGIE FAJITAS

Preparation Time: 15 min.   **Cooking Time:** 10 min.   **Servings**: 4

Ingredients:

- 3 large eggs
- 3 egg whites
- 2 tsp. chili powder
- 1 tbsp. unsalted butter
- 1 onion, chopped
- 2 garlic cloves, minced
- 1 jalapeño pepper, minced
- 1 red bell pepper, chopped
- 1 cup frozen corn, thawed and drained
- 8 (6-inch) corn tortillas

Directions:

1. Whisk the eggs, egg whites, and chili powder in a small bowl until well combined. Set aside.
2. Prepare a large skillet and melt the butter on medium heat.
3. Sauté the onion, garlic, jalapeño, bell pepper, and corn until the vegetables are tender, 3 to 4 min.
4. Add the beaten egg mixture to the skillet. Cook, occasionally stirring, until the eggs form large curds and are set, 3 to 5 min.
5. Meanwhile, soften the corn tortillas as directed on the package.
6. Divide the egg mixture evenly among the softened corn tortillas. Roll the tortillas up and serve.

Nutrition - Per Serving: Calories: 316; Fat 14g; Carbs: 35g; Protein: 14g; Sodium: 167mg; Potassium: 408mg; Phosphorus: 287mg

---

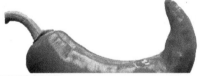

174.   VEGETABLE BIRYANI

Preparation Time: 10 min.   **Cooking Time:** 15 min.   **Servings**: 4

Ingredients:

- 2 tbsp. olive oil
- 1 onion, diced
- 4 garlic cloves, minced
- 1 tbsp. peeled and grated fresh ginger root
- 1 cup carrot, grated
- 2 cups chopped cauliflower
- 1 cup thawed frozen baby peas
- 2 tsp. curry powder
- 1 cup low-sodium vegetable broth
- 3 cups of frozen cooked brown rice

Directions:

1. Get a skillet and heat the olive oil on medium heat.
2. Add onion, garlic, and ginger root. Sauté, frequently stirring, until tender-crisp, 2 min.
3. Add the carrot, cauliflower, peas, and curry powder and cook for 2 min. longer.
4. Put vegetable broth. Cover the skillet partially, and simmer on low for 6 to 7 min. or until the vegetables are tender.
5. Meanwhile, heat the rice as directed on the package.
6. Stir the rice into the vegetable mixture and serve.
7.

Nutrition - Per Serving: Calories: 378; Fat 16g; Carbs: 53g; Protein: 8g; Sodium: 113mg; Potassium: 510mg; Phosphorus: 236mg

175.   PESTO PASTA SALAD

Preparation Time: 15 min.   **Cooking Time:** 15 min.   **Servings**: 4

Ingredients:

- 1 cup fresh basil leaves
- ½ cup packed fresh flat-leaf parsley leaves
- ½ cup arugula, chopped
- 2 tbsp. Parmesan cheese, grated
- ¼ cup extra-virgin olive oil
- 3 tbsp. mayonnaise
- 2 tbsp. water
- 12 ounces whole-wheat rotini pasta
- 1 red bell pepper, chopped
- 1 medium yellow summer squash, sliced
- 1 cup frozen baby peas

Directions:

1. Boil water in a large pot.
2. Meanwhile, combine the basil, parsley, arugula, cheese, and olive oil in a blender or food processor. Process until the herbs are finely chopped. Add the mayonnaise and water, then process again. Set aside.
3. Prepare the pasta to the pot of boiling water; cook according to package directions, about 8 to 9 min. Drain well, reserving ¼ cup of the cooking liquid.
4. Combine the pesto, pasta, bell pepper, squash, and peas in a large bowl and toss gently, adding enough reserved pasta cooking liquid to make a sauce on the salad. Serve immediately or cover and chill, then serve.
5. Store covered in the refrigerator for up to 3 days.

Nutrition - Per Serving: Calories: 378; Fat: 24g; Carbs: 35g; Protein: 9g; Sodium: 163mg; Potassium: 472mg; Phosphorus: 213mg

176.   BARLEY BLUEBERRY AVOCADO SALAD

Preparation Time: 15 min.   **Cooking Time:** 15 min.   **Servings**: 4

Ingredients:

- 1 cup quick-cooking barley
- 3 cups low-sodium vegetable broth
- 3 tbsp. extra-virgin olive oil
- 2 tbsp. freshly squeezed lemon juice
- 1 tsp. yellow mustard
- 1 tsp. honey
- ½ avocado, peeled and chopped
- 2 cups blueberries
- ¼ cup crumbled feta cheese

Directions:

1. Combine the barley and vegetable broth in a medium saucepan and bring to a simmer.
2. Reduce the heat to low, partially cover the pan, and simmer for 10 to 12 min. or until the barley is tender.
3. Meanwhile, whisk together the olive oil, lemon juice, mustard, and honey in a serving bowl until blended.Drain the barley if necessary and add to the bowl; toss to combine.
4. Add the avocado, blueberries, and feta and toss gently. Serve.

Nutrition - Per Serving: Calories: 345; Fat 16g; Carbs: 44g; Protein: 7g; Sodium: 259mg; Potassium: 301mg; Phosphorus: 152mg

177. PASTA WITH CREAMY BROCCOLI SAUCE

Preparation Time: 15 min. **Cooking Time:** 15 min. **Servings**: 4

Ingredients:

- 2 tbsp. olive oil
- 1-pound broccoli florets
- 3 garlic cloves, halved
- 1 cup low-sodium vegetable broth
- ½ pound whole-wheat spaghetti pasta
- 4 ounces cream cheese
- 1 tsp. dried basil leaves
- ½ cup grated Parmesan cheese

Directions:

1. Prepare a large pot of water to a boil.
2. Put olive oil in a large skillet. Sauté the broccoli and garlic for 3 min. Add the broth to the skillet and bring to a simmer. Reduce the heat to low, partially cover the skillet, and simmer until the broccoli is tender about 5 to 6 min.
3. Cook the pasta according to package directions. Drain when al dente, reserving 1 cup pasta water.
4. When the broccoli is tender, add the cream cheese and basil—purée using an immersion blender. Put mixture into a food processor, about half at a time, and purée until smooth and transfer the sauce back into the skillet.
5. Add the cooked pasta to the broccoli sauce. Toss, adding enough pasta water until the sauce coats the pasta completely. Sprinkle with the Parmesan and serve.

Nutrition - Per Serving: Calories: 302; Fat 14g; Carbs: 36g; Protein: 11g; Sodium: 260mg; Potassium: 375mg; Phosphorus: 223mg

178. ASPARAGUS FRIED RICE

Preparation Time: 10 min. **Cooking Time:** 10 min. **Servings**: 1

Ingredients:

- 3 large eggs, beaten
- ½ tsp. ground ginger
- 2 tsp. low-sodium soy sauce
- 2 tbsp. olive oil
- 1 onion, diced
- 4 garlic cloves, minced
- 1 cup sliced cremini mushrooms
- 1 (10-ounce) package frozen brown rice, thawed
- 8 ounces fresh asparagus, about 15 spears, cut into 1-inch pieces
- 1 tsp. sesame oil

Directions:

1. Whisk the eggs, ginger, and soy sauce in a small bowl and set aside.

2. Heat the olive oil in a medium skillet or wok over medium heat.
3. Add the onion and garlic and sauté for 2 min. until tender crisp.
4. Add the mushrooms and rice; stir-fry for 3 min. longer.
5. Put asparagus and cook for 2 min.6.
6. Pour in the egg mixture. Stir the eggs until cooked through, 2 to 3 min., and stir into the rice mixture.Sprinkle the fried rice with the sesame oil and serve.

Nutrition - Per Serving: Calories: 247; Fat: 13g; Carbs: 25g; Protein: 9g; Sodium: 149mg; Potassium: 367mg; Phosphorus: 206mg

179. VEGETARIAN TACO SALAD

Preparation Time: 15 min.   **Cooking Time:** 15 min.   **Servings**: 2

Ingredients:

- 1½ cups canned low-sodium or no-salt-added pinto beans, rinsed and drained
- 1 (10-ounce) package frozen brown rice, thawed
- 1 red bell pepper, chopped
- 3 scallions, white and green parts, chopped
- 1 jalapeño pepper, minced
- 1 cup frozen corn, thawed and drained
- 1 tbsp. chili powder
- 1 cup chopped romaine lettuce
- 2 cups chopped butter lettuce
- ½ cup Powerhouse Salsa
- ½ cup grated pepper Jack cheese

Directions:

1. In a medium bowl, combine the beans, rice, bell pepper, scallions, jalapeño, and corn.
2. Sprinkle with the chili powder and stir gently.
3. Stir in the romaine and butter lettuce.
4. Serve topped with Powerhouse Salsa and cheese.

Nutrition - Per Serving: Calories: 254; Fat: 7g; Carbs: 39g; Protein: 11g; Sodium: 440mg; Potassium: 599mg; Phosphorus: 240mg

180. SAUTÉED GREEN BEANS

Preparation Time: 10 min.   **Cooking Time:** 15 min.   **Servings**: 4

Ingredients:

- 2 cup frozen green beans
- ½ cup red bell pepper
- 4 tsp. margarine
- ¼ cup onion
- 1 tsp. dried dill weed
- 1 tsp. dried parsley
- ¼ tsp. black pepper

Directions:

1. Cook green beans in a large pan of boiling water until tender, then drain. While the beans are cooking, melt the margarine in a skillet and fry the other vegetables.
2. Add the beans to sautéed vegetables.
3. Sprinkle with freshly ground pepper and serve with meat and fish dishes.

Nutrition - Per Serving: Calories: 67; Carbs 8g: Protein 4g: Sodium 5mg; Potassium 179mg; Phosphorous 32mg

181. GARLICKY PENNE PASTA WITH ASPARAGUS

Preparation Time: 10 min.   **Cooking Time:** 10 min.   **Servings**: 4

Ingredients:

- 2 tbsp. butter
- 1lb asparagus, cut into 2-inch pieces
- 2 tsp. lemon juice

- 4 cup whole wheat penne pasta, cooked
- ¼ cup shredded Parmesan cheese
- ¼ tsp. Tabasco® hot sauce

Directions:

1. Add olive oil and butter in a skillet over medium heat.
2. Fry garlic and red pepper flakes for 2-3 min.
3. Add asparagus, Tabasco sauce, lemon juice, and black pepper to skillet and cook for a further 6 min.
4. Add hot pasta and cheese. Toss and serve.

Nutrition - Per Serving: Calories: 387; Carbs 49g; Protein 13g; Sodium 93mg; Potassium 258mg; Phosphorous 252mg

182.   GARLIC MASHED POTATOES

Preparation Time: 5 min.   **Cooking Time:** 20 min.   **Servings**: 4

Ingredients:

- 2 medium potatoes, peeled and sliced
- ¼ cup butter
- ¼ cup 1% low-fat milk
- 2 garlic cloves

Directions:

1. Double-boil or soak the potatoes to reduce potassium if you are on a low potassium diet.
2. Boil potatoes and garlic until soft. Drain.
3. Beat the potatoes and garlic with butter and milk until smooth.

Nutrition - Per Serving: Calories: 168: Carbs 29g; Protein 5g; Sodium 59 mg; Potassium 161 mg; Phosphorous 57mg

183.   GINGER GLAZED CARROTS

Preparation Time: 10 min.   **Cooking Time:** 20 min.   **Servings**: 4

Ingredients:

- 2 cups carrots, sliced into 1-inch pieces
- ¼ cup apple juice
- 2 tbsp. margarine, melted
- ¼ cup boiling water
- 1 tbsp. sugar
- 1 tsp. cornstarch
- ¼ tsp. salt
- ¼ tsp. ground ginger

Directions:

1. Cook carrots until tender.
2. Mix sugar, cornstarch, salt, ginger, apple juice, and margarine together
3. Pour mixture over carrots and cook for 10 min. until thickened.

Nutrition - Per Serving: Calories: 101; Fat 3; Carbs 14g; Protein 1g; Sodium 87 mg; Potassium 202 mg; Phosphorous 26mg

184.   CARROT-APPLE CASSEROLE

Preparation Time: 15 min.   **Cooking Time:** 50 min.   **Servings**: 8

Ingredients:

- 6 large carrots, peeled and sliced
- 4 large apples, peeled and sliced
- 3 tbsp. butter
- ½ cup apple juice
- 5 tbsp. all-purpose flour
- 2 tbsp. brown sugar
- ½ tsp. ground nutmeg

Directions:

1. Preheat oven to 350° F.
2. Let the carrots boil for 5 min. or until tender. Drain.

3. Arrange the carrots and apples in a large casserole dish.
4. Mix the flour, brown sugar, and nutmeg in a small bowl. Rub in butter to make a crumb topping.
5. Sprinkle the crumb over the carrots and apples, then drizzle with juice. Bake until bubbling and golden brown.

Nutrition - Per Serving: Calories: 245; Fat 6g; Carbs 49g; Protein 1g; Sodium 91mg; Potassium 169mg; Phosphorous 17mg

185.   CREAMY SHELLS WITH PEAS AND BACON

Preparation Time: 15 min.   **Cooking Time:** 15 min.   **Servings**: 4

Ingredients:

- 1 cup part-skim ricotta cheese
- ½ cup grated Parmesan cheese
- 3 slices bacon, cut into strips
- 1 cup onion, chopped
- ¾ cup of frozen green peas
- 1 tbsp. olive oil
- ¼ tsp. black pepper
- 3 garlic cloves, minced
- 3 cup cooked whole-wheat small shell pasta
- 1 tbsp. lemon juice
- 2 tbsp. unsalted butter

Directions:

1. Place ricotta, Parmesan cheese, butter, and pepper in a large bowl.
2. Cook bacon in a skillet until crisp. Set aside.
3. Add the garlic and onion to the same skillet and fry until soft. Add to bowl with ricotta.
4. Cook the peas and add to the ricotta.
5. Add half a cup of the reserved cooking water and lemon juice to the ricotta mixture and mix well.
6. Add the pasta, bacon, and peas to the bowl and mix well. Put freshly ground black pepper and serve.

Nutrition - Per Serving: Calories: 429; Fat 14g; Carbs 27g; Protein 13g; Sodium 244mg; Potassium 172mg; Phosphorous 203mg

186.   DOUBLE-BOILED STEWED POTATOES

Preparation Time: 20 min.   **Cooking Time:** 30 min.   **Servings**: 4

Ingredients:

- 2 cup potatoes, diced into ½ inch cubes
- ½ cup hot water
- ½ cup liquid non-dairy creamer
- ¼ tsp. garlic powder
- ¼ tsp. black pepper
- 2 tbsp. margarine
- 2 tsp. all-purpose white flour

Directions:

1. Soak or double boil the potatoes if you are on a low potassium diet. Boil potatoes for 15 min.
2. Drain potatoes and return to pan. Add half a cup of hot water, the creamer, garlic powder, pepper, and margarine. Heat to a boil.
3. Mix the flour with a tbsp. of water and then stir this into the potatoes. Cook for 3 min. until the mixture has thickened and the flour has cooked

Nutrition - Per Serving: Calories: 184; Carbs 25g; Protein 2g; Sodium 72mg; Potassium 161mg; Phosphorous 65mg

187.   Double-Boiled Country Style Fried Potatoes

Preparation Time: 20 min.   **Cooking Time:** 20 min.   **Servings**: 4

Ingredients:

- 2 medium potatoes, cut into large chips
- ½ cup canola oil
- ¼ tsp. ground cumin
- ¼ tsp. paprika
- ¼ tsp. white pepper
- 3 tbsp. ketchup

Directions:

1. Soak or double boil the potatoes if you are on a low potassium diet.
2. Heat oil over medium heat in a skillet.
3. Fry the potatoes for around 10 min. until golden brown.
4. Drain potatoes, then sprinkle with cumin, pepper, and paprika.
5. Serve with ketchup or mayo.

Nutrition - Per Serving: Calories: 156; Fat 0.1g; Carbs 21g; Protein 2g; Sodium 3mg; Potassium 296mg: Phosphorous 34mg

188.   BROCCOLI-ONION LATKES

Preparation Time: 15 min.   **Cooking Time:** 20 min.   **Servings**: 4

Ingredients:

- 3 cups broccoli florets, diced
- ½ cup onion, chopped
- 2 large eggs, beaten
- 2 tbsp. all-purpose white flour
- 2 tbsp. olive oil

Directions:

1. Cook the broccoli for around 5 min. until tender. Drain. Mix the flour into the eggs.
2. Combine the onion, broccoli, and egg mixture and stir through.
3. Prepare olive oil in a skillet on medium-high heat. Drop a spoon of the mixture onto the pan to make 4 latkes.
4. Cook each side until golden brown. Drain on a paper towel and serve.

Nutrition - Per Serving: Calories: 140; Fat 0g; Carbs 7g; Protein 6g; Sodium 58mg; Potassium 276mg; Phosphorous 101mg

189.   CRANBERRY CABBAGE

Preparation Time: 10 min.   **Cooking Time:** 20 min.   **Servings**: 8

Ingredients:

- 10 ounces canned whole-berry cranberry sauce
- 1 tbsp. fresh lemon juice
- 1 medium head red cabbage
- 1/4 tsp. ground cloves

Directions:

1. Place the cranberry sauce, lemon juice, and cloves in a large pan and bring to the boil.
2. Add the cabbage and reduce it to a simmer.
3. Cook until the cabbage is tender, occasionally stirring to make sure the sauce does not stick.
4. Delicious served with beef, lamb, or pork.

Nutrition - Per Serving: Calories: 73; Fat 0g; Carbs 18g; Protein 1g; Sodium 32mg; Potassium 138mg; Phosphorous 18mg

190.   CAULIFLOWER RICE

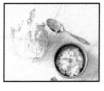

Preparation Time: 5 min.

Cooking Time: 10 min.

Servings: 1

Ingredients:

- 1 small head cauliflower cut into florets
- 1 tbsp. butter
- ¼ tsp. black pepper
- ¼ tsp. garlic powder
- ¼ tsp. salt-free herb seasoning blend

Directions:

1. Blitz cauliflower pieces in a food processor until it has a grain-like consistency.
2. Melt butter in a saucepan and add spices.
3. Add the cauliflower rice grains and cook over low-medium heat for approximately 10 min.
4. Use a fork to fluff the rice before serving.
5. Serve as an alternative to rice with curries, stews, and starch to accompany meat and fish dishes.

Nutrition - Per Serving: Calories: 47; Fat: 11.8g; Carbs: 4g; Protein :1g; Sodium: 300mg; Potassium: 206mg; Phosphorous: 31mg

191.   THAI TOFU BROTH

Preparation time: 5 min.   **Cooking time:** 15 min.   **Servings:** 4

Ingredients:

- 1 cup rice noodles
- ½ sliced onion
- 6 ounces drained, pressed and cubed tofu
- ¼ cup sliced scallions
- ½ cup water
- 200 grams water chestnuts
- ½ cup rice milk
- 1 tbsp.. coconut oil
- ½ finely sliced chili
- 1 cup snow peas

Directions:

1. Heat the oil and then sauté the tofu until brown on each side.
2. Add the onion and sauté for 2–3 min.
3. Add the rice milk and water to the wok until bubbling.
4. Lower to medium heat and add the noodles, chili, and water chestnuts.
5. Simmer for 15 min., and then add the sugar and peas for 5 min.
6. Serve with a sprinkle of scallions.

Nutrition: Calories: 304 Protein: 9g Carbs: 38g Fat 13g Sodium (Na): 36mg Potassium (K): 114mg Phosphorus: 101mg

192.   VEGETARIAN LASAGNA

Preparation time: 10 min.   **Cooking time**: 1 h.   **Servings:** 4

Ingredients:

- 1 tsp. basil
- 1 tbsp. olive oil
- ½ sliced red pepper
- 3 lasagna sheets
- ½ diced red onion
- ¼ tsp.. black pepper
- 1 cup rice milk
- 1 minced garlic clove
- 1 cup sliced eggplant
- ½ sliced zucchini
- ½ pack soft tofu
- 1 tsp. oregano

Directions:

1. Preheat oven to 325°F.
2. Slice zucchini, eggplant, and pepper into vertical strips.
3. Add the rice milk and tofu to a food processor and blitz until smooth. Set aside.
4. Sauté the onions and garlic until soft.
5. Sprinkle in the herbs and pepper and allow to stir through for 5–6 min. until hot.
6. Into a lasagna or suitable oven dish, layer 1 lasagna sheet, then 1/3 the eggplant, followed by 1/3 zucchini, then 1/3 pepper before pouring over 1/3 of white tofu sauce.
7. Repeat for the next 2 layers, finishing with the white sauce.
8. Add to the oven for 40–50 min. or until veg is soft and easily be sliced into servings.

Nutrition: Calories: 235 Protein: 5g Carbs: 10g Fat: 9g Sodium (Na): 35mg Potassium (K): 129mg Phosphorus: 66mg

193.   CHILI TOFU NOODLES

Preparation time: 5 min.   **Cooking time:** 15 min.   **Servings:** 4

Ingredients:

- ½ diced red chili
- 2 cups rice noodles
- ½ juiced lime
- 6 ounces pressed and cubed silken firm tofu

- 1 tsp.. grated fresh ginger
- 1 tbsp.. coconut oil
- 1 cup green beans
- 1 minced garlic clove

Directions:
1. Steam the green beans for 10–12 min. or according to package directions and drain.
2. Cook the noodles in a pot of boiling water for 10–15 min. or according to package directions. Meanwhile, heat a wok or skillet on high heat and add coconut oil.
3. Now add the tofu, chili flakes, garlic, and ginger and sauté for 5–10 min.
4. Drain the noodles.
5. Add to the wok along with the green beans and lime juice. Toss to coat.
6. Serve hot!

Nutrition: Calories: 246 Protein: 10g Carbs: 28g Fat: 12g Sodium (Na): 25mg Potassium (K): 126mg Phosphorus: 79mg

194. CURRIED CAULIFLOWER

Preparation time: 5 min.   **Cooking time**: 20 min.   **Servings**: 4

Ingredients:
- 1 tsp.. turmeric
- 1 diced onion
- 1 tbsp. chopped fresh cilantro
- 1 tsp.. cumin
- ½ diced chili
- ½ cup water
- 1 minced garlic clove
- 1 tbsp.. coconut oil
- 1 tsp.. garam masala
- 2 cups cauliflower florets

Directions:
1. Heat the oil.
2. Sauté the onion and garlic for 5 min. until soft.
3. Add the turmeric, cumin and garam masala and stir to release the aromas.
4. Now add the chili to the pan along with the cauliflower. Stir to coat.
5. Pour in the water and reduce the heat to a simmer for 15 min.
6. Garnish with cilantro to serve.

Nutrition: Calories: 108 Protein: 2g Carbs: 11g Fat: 7g Sodium (Na): 35mg Potassium (K): 328mg Phosphorus: 39mg

195. BROCCOLI PANCAKE

Preparation time: 10 min.   **Cooking time**: 5 min.   **Servings**: 4

Ingredients:
- 3 cups broccoli florets, diced
- 2 eggs, beaten
- 2 tbsp. all-purpose flour
- 1/2 cup onion, chopped
- 2 tbsp. olive oil

Directions:
1. Boil broccoli in water for 5 min. Drain and set aside.
2. Mix egg and flour.
3. Add onion and broccoli to the mixture.
4. Cook the broccoli pancake until brown on both sides.

Nutrition: Calories: 140 Protein: 6g Carbs: 7g Fat: 10g Cholesterol: 106mg Sodium: 58mg Potassium: 276mg Phosphorus: 101mg Calcium: 50mg Fiber: 2.1g

196. EGGPLANT FRIES

Preparation time: 10 min.   **Cooking time**: 5 min.   **Servings**: 6

Ingredients:
- 2 eggs, beaten
- 1 cup almond milk
- 1 tsp. hot sauce
- 3/4 cup cornstarch
- 3 tsp. dry ranch seasoning mix
- 3/4 cup dry breadcrumbs
- 1 eggplant, sliced into strips
- 1/2 cup oil

Directions:
1. In a bowl, mix eggs, milk and hot sauce.
2. In a dish, mix cornstarch, seasoning and breadcrumbs.
3. Dip first the eggplant strips in the egg mixture.
4. Coat each strip with the cornstarch mixture.
5. Heat oil in medium heat.
6. Once hot, add the fries and cook for 3 min. or until golden.

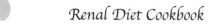

Nutrition: Calories: 234 Protein: 7g Carbs: 25g Fat: 13g Cholesterol: 48mg Sodium: 212mg Potassium: 215mg Phosphorus: 86mg Calcium: 70mg Fiber: 2.1g

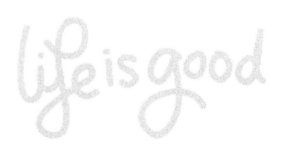

CHAPTER 10. POULTRY RECIPES

197.   ROASTED CITRUS CHICKEN

Preparation Time: 20mins   **Cooking Time:** 60mins   **Servings:** 8

Ingredients:

- 1 - tbsp. olive oil
- 2 - cloves garlic, minced
- 1 - tsp. Italian seasoning
- ½ - tsp. black pepper
- 8 - chicken thighs
- 2 - cups chicken broth, reduced-sodium
- 3 - tbsp. lemon juice
- ½ - large chicken breast for 1 chicken thigh

Directions:

1. Warm oil in colossal skillet.
2. Include garlic and seasonings.
3. Include chicken bosoms and dark-colored all sides.
4. Spot chicken in the moderate cooker and include the chicken soup. Cook on LOW heat for 6 to 8hs
5. Include lemon juice toward the part of the bargain time.

Nutrition - Per Serving: Calories: 265 Fat: 19g Protein: 21g Carbs: 1g Sodium: 453mg; Potassium: 404mg

---

198.   CHICKEN WITH ASIAN VEGETABLES

Preparation Time: 10mins   **Cooking Time:** 20mins   **Servings:** 8

Ingredients:

- 2 - tbsp. canola oil
- 6 - boneless chicken breasts
- 1 - cup low-sodium chicken broth
- 3 - tbsp. reduced-sodium soy sauce
- ¼ - tsp. crushed red pepper flakes
- 1 - garlic clove, crushed
- 1 - can (8ounces) water chestnuts, sliced and rinsed (optional)
- ½ - cup sliced green onions
- 1 - cup chopped red or green bell pepper
- 1 - cup chopped celery
- ¼ - cup cornstarch
- 1/3 - cup water
- 3 - cups cooked white rice
- ½ - large chicken breast for 1 chicken thigh

Directions:

1. Warm oil in a skillet and dark-colored chicken on all sides.
2. Add chicken to slow cooker with the remainder of the fixings aside from cornstarch and water. Spread and cook on LOW for 6 to 8hs
3. Following 6-8 hs, independently blend cornstarch and cold water until smooth. Gradually include into the moderate cooker.
4. At that point turn on high for about 15mins until thickened. Don't close top on the moderate cooker to enable steam to leave.
5. Serve Asian blend over rice.

Nutrition - Per Serving: Calories: 415; Fat: 20g; Protein: 20g; Carbs: 36g; Sodium 1176mg; Potassium 321mg

---

199.   CHICKEN ADOBO

Preparation Time: 10mins   **Cooking Time:** 1hr 40mins   **Servings:** 6

Ingredients:

- 4 - medium yellow onions, halved and thinly sliced
- 4 - medium garlic cloves, smashed and peeled
- 1 - (5-inch) piece fresh ginger, cut into
- 1 - inch pieces
- 1 - bay leaf

- 3 - pounds bone-in chicken thighs
- 3 - Tbsp. reduced-sodium soy sauce
- ¼ - cup rice vinegar (not seasoned)
- 1 - Tbsp. granulated sugar
- ½ - tsp. freshly ground black pepper

Directions:

1. Spot the onions, garlic, ginger, and narrows leaf in an even layer in the slight cooker.
2. Take out and do away with the pores and skin from the chicken.
3. Organize the hen in an even layer over the onion mixture.
4. Whisk the soy sauce, vinegar, sugar, and pepper collectively in a medium bowl and pour it over the fowl.
5. Spread and prepare dinner on LOW for 8hs
6. Evacuate and take away the ginger portions and inlet leaf. Present with steamed rice.

Nutrition - Per Serving: Calories:318; Fat: 9g; Protein: 14g; Carbs: 44g; Sodium: 392mg; Potassium: 128mg

200.   CHICKEN AND VEGGIE SOUP

Preparation Time: 15mins   **Cooking Time:** 25mins   **Servings**: 8

Ingredients:

- 4 - cups cooked and chopped chicken
- 7 - cups reduced-sodium chicken broth
- 1 - pound frozen white corn
- 1 - medium onion diced
- 4 - cloves garlic minced
- 2 - carrots peeled and diced
- 2 - celery stalks chopped
- 2 - tsp. oregano
- 2 - tsp. curry powder
- ½ - tsp. black pepper

Directions:

1. Include all fixings into the moderate cooker.
2. Cook on LOW for 8hs
3. Serve over cooked white rice.

Nutrition - Per Serving: Calories:220; Fat:7g; Protein: 24g; Carbs: 19g; Sodium: 751mg; Potassium: 448mg

201.   TURKEY SAUSAGES

Preparation Time: 10 Min.   **Cooking Time:** 10 min.   **Servings**: 2

Ingredients:

- 1/4 tsp. salt
- 1/8 tsp. garlic powder
- 1/8 tsp. onion powder
- 1 tsp. fennel seed
- 1 pound 7% fat ground turkey

Directions:

1. Press the fennel seed and put together turkey with fennel seed, garlic and onion powder, and salt in a small cup.
2. Cover the bowl and refrigerate overnight.
3. Prepare the turkey with seasoning into different portions with a circle form and press them into patties ready to be cooked.
4. Cook at a medium heat until browned.
5. Cook it for 1 to 2 min. per side and serve them hot. Enjoy!

Nutrition - Per Serving: Calories: 55; Protein: 7 g; Fat 0.3g; Carbs: 0.8g; Sodium: 70 mg; Potassium: 105 mg; Phosphorus: 75 mg.

202.   ROSEMARY CHICKEN

Preparation Time: 10 Min.   **Cooking Time:** 10 min.   **Servings**: 2

Ingredients:

- 2 zucchinis
- 1 carrot
- 1 tsp. dried rosemary
- 4 chicken breasts
- 1/2 bell pepper
- 1/2 red onion
- 8 garlic cloves
- Olive oil
- 1/4 tbsp. ground pepper

Directions:

1. Prepare the oven and preheat it at 375 °F (or 200°C). Slice both zucchini and carrots and add bell pepper, onion, garlic and put everything adding oil in a 13" x 9" pan.
2. Spread the pepper over everything and roast for about 10 min.
3. Meanwhile, lift the chicken skin and spread black pepper and rosemary on the flesh.
4. Remove the vegetable pan from the oven and add the chicken, returning it to the oven for about 30 more min. Serve and enjoy!

Nutrition - Per Serving: Calories: 215; Protein: 28 g; Fat 11.5g; Carbs: 19.3g; Sodium: 105 mg Potassium: 580 mg Phosphorus: 250 mg

203.   SMOKY TURKEY CHILI

Preparation Time: 5 min.   **Cooking Time:** 45 min.   **Servings**: 8

Ingredients:

- 12ounce lean ground turkey
- 1/2 red onion, chopped
- 2 cloves garlic, crushed and chopped
- ½ tsp. of smoked paprika
- ½ tsp. of chili powder
- ½ tsp. of dried thyme
- ¼ cup reduced-sodium beef stock
- ½ cup of water
- 1 ½ cups baby spinach leaves, washed
- 3 wheat tortillas

Directions:

1. Brown the ground beef in a dry skillet over a medium-high heat.
2. Add in the red onion and garlic.
3. Sauté the onion until it goes clear.
4. Transfer the contents of the skillet to the slow cooker. Add the remaining ingredients and simmer on Low for 30–45 min.
5. Stir through the spinach for the last few min. to wilt.
6. Slice tortillas and gently toast under the broiler until slightly crispy. Serve on top of the turkey chili.

Nutrition - Per Serving: Calories: 93.5 Protein: 8g Carbs: 3g Fat: 5.5g Cholesterol: 30.5mg Sodium: 84.5mg Potassium: 142.5mg Phosphorus: 92.5mgCalcium: 29mg Fiber: 0.5g

204.   AVOCADO-ORANGE GRILLED CHICKEN

Preparation Time: 20 min.   **Cooking Time:** 60 min.   **Servings**: 4

Ingredients:

- ¼ cup fresh lime juice
- ¼ cup minced red onion
- 1 avocado
- 1 cup low fat yogurt
- 1 small red onion, sliced thinly
- 1 tbsp. honey
- 2 oranges, peeled and sectioned
- 2 tbsp. chopped cilantro
- 4 pieces of 4-6ounce boneless, skinless chicken breasts
- Pepper and salt to taste

Directions:

1. In a large bowl mix honey, cilantro, minced red onion and yogurt. Submerge chicken into mixture and marinate for at least 30 min.
2. Grease grate and preheat grill to medium high fire. Remove chicken from marinade and season with pepper and salt.
3. Grill for 6 min. per side or until chicken is cooked and juices run clear.

4. Meanwhile, peel avocado and discard seed. Chop avocados and place in bowl. Quickly add lime juice and toss avocado to coat well with liquid.
5. Add cilantro, thinly sliced onions and oranges into bowl of avocado, mix well.
6. Serve grilled chicken and avocado dressing on the side.

Nutrition - Per Serving: Calories: per Serving: 209; Carbs: 26g; protein: 8g; fats: 10g; phosphorus: 157mg; potassium: 548mg; sodium: 125mg

205. HERBS AND LEMONY ROASTED CHICKEN

Preparation Time: 15 min.   **Cooking Time:** 1 ½ hs   **Servings**: 8

Ingredients:

- ½ tsp. ground black pepper
- ½ tsp. mustard powder
- ½ tsp. salt
- 1 3-lb whole chicken
- 1 tsp. garlic powder
- 2 lemons
- 2 tbsp. olive oil
- 2 tsp.. Italian seasoning

Directions:

1. In small bowl, mix well black pepper, garlic powder, mustard powder, and salt.
2. Rinse chicken well and slice off giblets.
3. In a greased 9 x 13 baking dish, place chicken and add 1 ½ tsp.. of seasoning made earlier inside the chicken and rub the remaining seasoning around chicken.

4. In small bowl, mix olive oil and juice from 2 lemons. Drizzle over chicken.
5. Bake chicken in a preheated 350 F oven until juices run clear, around 1 ½ hs. Every once in a while, baste chicken with its juices

Nutrition - Per Serving: Calories: per Serving: 190; Carbs: 2g; protein: 35g; fats: 9g; phosphorus: 341mg; potassium: 439mg; sodium: 328mg

206. GROUND CHICKEN & PEAS CURRY

Preparation Time: 15 min.   **Cooking Time:** 6-10 min.   **Servings**: 3-4

Ingredients:

FOR MARINADE:

- 3 tbsp. essential olive oil
- 2 bay leaves
- 2 onions, grinded to some paste
- ½ tbsp. garlic paste
- ½ tbsp. ginger paste
- 2 tomatoes, chopped finely
- 1 tbsp. ground cumin
- 1 tbsp. ground coriander
- 1 tsp. ground turmeric
- 1 tsp. red chili powder
- Salt, to taste
- 1-pound lean ground chicken
- 2 cups frozen peas
- 1½ cups water
- 1-2 tsp. garam masala powder

Directions:

1. In a deep skillet, heat oil on medium heat.
2. Add bay leaves and sauté for approximately half a min. Add onion paste and sauté for approximately 3-4 min.
3. Add garlic and ginger paste and sauté for around 1-1½ min.

4. Add tomatoes and spices and cook, stirring occasionally for about 3-4 min.
5. Stir in chicken and cook for about 4-5 min.
6. Stir in peas and water and bring to a boil on high heat. Reduce the heat to low and simmer approximately 5-8 min. or till desired doneness. Stir in garam masala and remove from heat.

7. Serve hot.

Nutrition - Per Serving: Calories: 450, Fat: 10g, Carbs: 19g, Fiber: 6g, Protein: 38g; Sodium: 247mg; Potassium: 387mg

207. CHICKEN MEATBALLS CURRY

Preparation Time: 20 min   **Cooking Time:** 25 min.   **Servings**: 3-4

Ingredients:

FOR MEATBALLS:

- 1-pound lean ground chicken
- 1 tbsp. onion paste
- 1 tsp. fresh ginger paste
- 1 tsp. garlic paste
- 1 green chili, chopped finely
- 1 tbsp. fresh cilantro leaves, chopped
- 1 tsp. ground coriander
- ½ tsp. cumin seeds
- ½ tsp. red chili powder
- ½ tsp. ground turmeric

- Salt, to taste

FOR CURRY:

- 3 tbsp. extra-virgin olive oil
- ½ tsp. cumin seeds
- 1 (1-inch) cinnamon stick
- 3 whole cloves
- 3 whole green cardamoms
- 1 whole black cardamom
- 2 onions, chopped
- 1 tsp. fresh ginger, minced
- 1 tsp. garlic, minced

- 4 whole tomatoes, chopped finely
- 2 tsp. ground coriander
- 1 tsp. garam masala powder
- ½ tsp. ground nutmeg
- ½ tsp. red chili powder
- ½ tsp. ground turmeric
- Salt, to taste
- 1 cup water
- Chopped fresh cilantro, for garnishing

Directions:

1. For meatballs in a substantial bowl, add all ingredients and mix till well combined.
2. Make small equal-sized meatballs from mixture. In a big deep skillet, heat oil on medium heat. Add meatballs and fry approximately 3-5 min. or till browned from all sides. Transfer the meatballs in a bowl.
3. In the same skillet, add cumin seeds, cinnamon stick, cloves, green cardamom and black cardamom and sauté approximately 1 min.
4. Add onions and sauté for around 4-5 min.
5. Add ginger and garlic paste and sauté approximately 1 min.
6. Add tomato and spices and cook, crushing with the back of spoon for approximately 2-3 min.
7. Add water and meatballs and provide to a boil.
8. Reduce heat to low.
9. Simmer for approximately 10 min.
10. Serve hot with all the garnishing of cilantro.

Nutrition - Per Serving: Calories: 421, Fat: 8g, Carbs: 18g, Fiber: 5g, Protein: 34g; Sodium: 213mg; Potassium: 434mg

208. GROUND CHICKEN WITH BASIL

Preparation Time: f15 min.   **Cooking Time:** 16 min.   **Servings**: 8

Ingredients:

- 2 pounds lean ground chicken
- 3 tbsp. coconut oil, divided
- 1 zucchini, chopped
- 1 red bell pepper, seeded and chopped
- ½ of green bell pepper, seeded and chopped
- 4 garlic cloves, minced
- 1 (1-inch) piece fresh ginger, minced
- 1 (1-inch) piece fresh turmeric, minced

- 1 fresh red chile, sliced thinly
- 1 tbsp. organic honey
- 1 tbsp. coconut amino
- 1½ tbsp. fish sauce
- ½ cup fresh basil, chopped
- Salt and freshly ground black pepper, to taste
- 1 tbsp. fresh lime juice

Directions:

1. Heat a large skillet on medium-high heat.

2. Add ground beef and cook for approximately 5 min. or till browned completely. Transfer the beef in a bowl.
3. In a similar pan, melt 1 tbsp. of coconut oil on medium-high heat.
4. Add zucchini and bell peppers and stir fry for around 3-4 min.
5. Transfer the vegetables inside bowl with chicken.

6. In exactly the same pan, melt remaining coconut oil on medium heat.
7. Add garlic, ginger, turmeric and red chile and sauté for approximately 1-2 min.
8. Add chicken mixture, honey and coconut amino and increase the heat to high.
9. Cook, stirring occasionally for approximately 4-5 min. or till sauce is nearly reduced.
10. Stir in remaining ingredients and take off from heat.

Nutrition - Per Serving: Calories: 407, Fat: 7g, Carbs: 20g, Fiber: 13g, Protein: 36g; Sodium: 113mg; Potassium: 207mg

209.   CHICKEN &VEGGIE CASSEROLE

Preparation Time: 15 min.   **Cooking Time:** half an h   **Servings**: 4

Ingredients:

- 1/3 cup Dijon mustard
- 1/3 cup organic honey
- 1 tsp. dried basil
- ¼ tsp. ground turmeric
- 1 tsp. dried basil, crushed

- Salt and freshly ground black pepper, to taste
- 1¾ pound chicken breasts
- 1 cup fresh white mushrooms, sliced
- ½ head broccoli, cut into small florets

Directions:

1. Preheat the oven to 350 F. Lightly, grease a baking dish.
2. In a bowl, mix all ingredients except chicken, mushrooms and broccoli.
3. Arrange chicken in prepared baking dish and top with mushroom slices.

4. Place broccoli florets around chicken evenly.
5. Pour 1 / 2 of honey mixture over chicken and broccoli evenly.
6. Bake for approximately twenty min.
7. Now, coat the chicken with remaining sauce and bake for approximately 10 min.

Nutrition - Per Serving: Calories: 427, Fat: 9g, Carbs: 16g, Fiber: 7g, Protein: 35g; Sodium: 559mg; Potassium: 1035mg

210.   CHICKEN & CAULIFLOWER RICE CASSEROLE

Preparation Time: 15min.   **Cooking Time:** 1h 15 min.   **Servings**: 8-10

Ingredients:

- 2 tbsp. coconut oil, divided
- 3-pound bone-in chicken thighs and drumsticks
- Salt and freshly ground black pepper, to taste
- 3 carrots, peeled and sliced
- 1 onion, chopped finely
- 2 garlic cloves, chopped finely
- 2 tbsp. fresh cinnamon, chopped finely

- 2 tsp. ground cumin
- 1 tsp. ground coriander
- 12 tsp. ground cinnamon
- ½ tsp. ground turmeric
- 1 tsp. paprika
- ¼ tsp. red pepper cayenne
- 1 (28-ounce) can diced tomatoes with liquid
- 1 red bell pepper, seeded and cut into thin strips

- ½ cup fresh parsley leaves, minced
- Salt, to taste
- 1 head cauliflower, grated to some rice like consistency
- 1 lemon, sliced thinly

Directions:

1. Preheat the oven to 375 F.

2. In a large pan, melt 1 tbsp. of coconut oil high heat. Add chicken pieces and cook for about 3-5 min. per side or till golden brown.
3. Transfer the chicken in a plate.
4. In a similar pan, sauté the carrot, onion, garlic and ginger for about 4-5 min. on medium heat. Stir in spices and remaining coconut oil.
5. Add chicken, tomatoes, bell pepper, parsley and salt and simmer for approximately 3-5 min.

In the bottom of a 13x9-inch rectangular baking dish, spread the cauliflower rice evenly.
6. Place chicken mixture over cauliflower rice evenly and top with lemon slices.
7. With a foil paper, cover the baking dish and bake for approximately 35 min.
8. Uncover the baking dish and bake approximately 25 min.

Nutrition - Per Serving: Calories: 412, Fat: 12g, Carbs: 23g, Fiber: 7g, Protein: 34g; Sodium: 849mg; Phosphorus: mg; Potassium: 219mg

211. CHICKEN MEATLOAF WITH VEGGIES

Preparation Time: 20 min.   **Cooking Time:** 1-1¼ hs   **Servings:** 4

Ingredients:

FOR MEATLOAF:
- ½ cup cooked chickpeas
- 2 egg whites
- 2½ tsp. poultry seasoning
- Salt and freshly ground black pepper, to taste
- 10-ounce lean ground chicken
- 1 cup red bell pepper, seeded and minced
- 1 cup celery stalk, minced
- 1/3 cup steel-cut oats
- 1 cup tomato puree, divided
- 2 tbsp. dried onion flakes, crushed
- 1 tbsp. prepared mustard

FOR VEGGIES:
- 2-pounds summer squash, sliced
- 16-ounce frozen Brussels sprouts
- 2 tbsp. extra-virgin extra virgin olive oil
- Salt and freshly ground black pepper, to taste

Directions:

1. Preheat the oven to 350 F. Grease a 9x5-inch loaf pan. In a mixer, add chickpeas, egg whites, poultry seasoning, salt and black pepper and pulse till smooth. Transfer a combination in a large bowl.
2. Add chicken, veggies oats, ½ cup of tomato puree and onion flakes and mix till well combined.
3. Transfer the amalgamation into prepared loaf pan evenly.
4. With both hands, press, down the amalgamation slightly. In another bowl mix together mustard and remaining tomato puree.
5. Place the mustard mixture over loaf pan evenly. Bake approximately 1-1¼ hs or till desired doneness.
6. Meanwhile in a big pan of water, arrange a steamer basket.
7. Bring to a boil and set summertime squash I steamer basket. Cover and steam approximately 10-12 min. Drain well and aside. Now, prepare the Brussels sprouts according to package's directions.
8. In a big bowl, add veggies, oil, salt and black pepper and toss to coat well. Serve the meatloaf with veggies.

Nutrition: Calories: 420, Fat: 9g, Carbs: 21g, Fiber: 14g, Protein: 36g; Sodium: 220mg; Potassium: 1673mg

212. ROASTED SPATCHCOCK CHICKEN

Preparation Time: 20 min.   **Cooking Time:** 50 min.   **Servings:** 4-6

Ingredients:
- 1 (4-pound) whole chicken
- 1 (1-inch) piece fresh ginger, sliced
- 4 garlic cloves, chopped
- 1 small bunch fresh thyme
- Pinch of cayenne
- Salt and freshly ground black pepper, to taste
- ¼ cup fresh lemon juice
- 3 tbsp. extra-virgin olive oil

Directions:

1. Arrange chicken, breast side down onto a large cutting board.
2. With a kitchen shear, begin with thigh and cut along 1 side of backbone and turn chicken around. Now, cut along sleep issues and discard the backbone. Change the inside and open it like a book. Flatten the backbone firmly to flatten.
3. In a food processor, add all ingredients except chicken and pulse till smooth.
4. In a big baking dish, add the marinade mixture.
5. Add chicken and coat with marinade generously. With a plastic wrap, cover the baking dish and refrigerate to marinate for overnight.
6. Preheat the oven to 450 F. Arrange a rack in a very roasting pan.
7. Remove the chicken from refrigerator make onto rack over roasting pan, skin side down.
8. Roast for about 50 min., turning once in the middle way.

Nutrition: Calories: 419, Fat: 14g, Carbs: 28g, Fiber: 4g, Protein: 40g; Sodium: 454mg; Potassium: 1673mg

213.   CREAMY MUSHROOM AND BROCCOLI CHICKEN

Preparation Time: 15 min.   **Cooking Time:** 6 hs   **Servings**: 6

Ingredients:

- 1 10.5 ounce can of low-sodium cream of mushroom soup
- 1 21 ounce can of low-sodium cream of Chicken Soup
- 2 whole cooked chicken breasts, chopped or shredded
- 2 cup milk
- 1lb broccoli florets
- ¼ tsp. garlic powder

Directions:

1. Place all ingredients to a 5 quart or larger slow cooker and mix well.
2. Cover and cook on LOW for 6 hs.
3. Serve with potatoes, pasta, or rice.

Nutrition - Per Serv: Calories: 155; Fat 2g; Carbs 19g, Protein 12g, Fiber 2g, Potassium 755mg, Sodium 35mg

214.   CHICKEN CURRY

Preparation Time: 10 min.   **Cooking Time:** 4 min.   **Servings**: 4

Ingredients:

- 1lb skinless chicken breasts
- 1 medium onion, thinly sliced
- 1 15 ounce can chickpeas, drained and rinsed well
- 2 medium sweet potatoes, peeled and diced
- ½ cup light coconut milk
- ½ cup chicken stock (see recipe)
- 1 15ounce can sodium-free tomato sauce
- 2 tbsp. curry powder
- 1 tsp. low-sodium salt
- ½ cayenne powder
- 1 cup green peas
- 2 tbsp. lemon juice

Directions:

1. Place the chicken breasts, onion, chickpeas, and sweet potatoes into a 4 to 6-quart slow cooker. Mix the coconut milk, chicken stock, tomato sauce, curry powder, salt, and cayenne and pour into the slow cooker, stirring to coat well.
2. Cover and cook on Low for 8 hs or High for 4 hs.
3. Stir in the peas and lemon juice 5 min. before serving.

Nutrition: Calories: 302, Fat 5g, Carbs 43g, Protein 24g, Fiber 9g, Potassium 573mg, Sodium 800mg.

215. APPLE & CINNAMON SPICED HONEY PORK LOIN

Preparation Time: 20 min.   **Cooking Time:** 6 hs   **Servings:** 6

Ingredients:

- 1 2-3lb boneless pork loin roast
- ½ tsp. low-sodium salt
- ¼ tsp. pepper
- 1 tbsp. canola oil
- 3 medium apples, peeled and sliced
- ¼ cup honey
- 1 small red onion, halved and sliced
- 1 tbsp. ground cinnamon

Directions:

1. Season the pork with salt and pepper.
2. Heat the oil in a skillet and brown the pork on all sides. Arrange half the apples in the base of a 4 to 6-quart slow cooker.
3. Top with the honey and remaining apples.
4. Sprinkle with cinnamon and cover.
5. Cover and cook on low for 6-8 hs until the meat is tender.

Nutrition: Calories: 290, Fat 10g, Carbs 19g, Protein 29g, Fiber 2g, Potassium 789mg, Sodium 22mg;

---

216. LEMON & HERB TURKEY BREASTS

Preparation Time: 25 min.   **Cooking Time:** 3 1/2 hs   **Servings:** 12

Ingredients:

- 1 can (14-1/2 ounces) chicken broth
- 1/2 cup lemon juice
- 1/4 cup packed brown sugar
- 1/4 cup fresh sage
- 1/4 cup fresh thyme leaves
- 1/4 cup lime juice
- 1/4 cup cider vinegar
- 1/4 cup olive oil
- 1 envelope low-sodium onion soup mix
- 2 tbsp. Dijon mustard
- 1 tbsp. fresh marjoram, minced
- 1 tsp. paprika
- 1 tsp. garlic powder
- 1 tsp. pepper
- ½ tsp. low-sodium salt
- 2 2lb boneless skinless turkey breast halves

Directions:

1. Make a marinade by blending all the ingredients in a blender.
2. Pour over the turkey and leave overnight.
3. Place the turkey and marinade in a 4 to 6-quart slow cooker and cover.
4. Cover and cook on HIGH for 3-1/2 to 4-1/2 hs or until a thermometer reads 165°.

Nutrition- Per Serv.: Calories: 219, Fat 5g, Carbs 3g, Protein 36g, Fiber 0g, Potassium 576mg, Sodium 484mg

---

217. BEEF CHIMICHANGAS

Preparation Time: 10min.   **Cooking Time:** 10-12 hs   **Servings:** 16

Ingredients:

- Shredded beef
- 3lb boneless beef chuck roast, fat trimmed away
- 3 tbsp. low-sodium taco seasoning mix
- 1 10ounce canned low-sodium diced tomatoes
- 6ounce canned diced green chilies with the juice
- 3 garlic cloves, minced
- To serve
- 16 medium flour tortillas
- Sodium-free refried beans
- Mexican rice, sour cream, cheddar cheese
- Guacamole, salsa, lettuce

Directions:

1. Arrange the beef in a 5-quart or larger slow cooker.
2. Sprinkle over taco seasoning and coat well.
3. Add tomatoes and garlic and cover.
4. Cook on low for 10 to 12 hs.
5. When cooked remove the beef and shred.
6. Make burritos out of the shredded beef, refried beans, Mexican rice, and cheese.
7. Bake for 10 min. at 350° f until brown.
8. Serve with salsa, lettuce, and guacamole.

Nutrition - Per Serv.: Calories: 249, fat 18g, Carbs 3g, Protein 33g, fiber 5g, Potassium 633mg, Sodium 457mg

218.   MEAT LOAF

Preparation Time: 5 min.   **Cooking Time:** 5-6 hs   **Servings**: 6

Ingredients:

- 2-pound lean ground beef
- 2 whole eggs, beaten
- ¾ cup milk
- ¾ cup breadcrumbs
- ½ cup chicken broth (see recipe)
- ¼ cup onion, finely diced
- 3 garlic cloves, minced
- 1 tsp. low-sodium salt
- ¼ tsp. freshly ground black pepper
- ¼ cup low sodium chili sauce
- Nonstick spray

Directions:

1. Mix the beaten eggs, milk, oatmeal, spices, onion, garlic, and chicken broth until well combined.
2. Mix in the beef and place in a 5-quart or larger slow cooker, sprayed with nonstick spray.
3. Cover and cook on low for 5 to 6 hs.
4. Serve with low-sodium ketchup.

Nutrition - Per Serv.: Calories: 280, fat 10g, Carbs 9g, protein 37g, fiber 1g, Potassium 648mg, Sodium 325mg

219.   CROCKPOT PEACHY PORK CHOPS

Preparation Time: 30min.   **Cooking Time:** 2-3 hs   **Servings**: 8

Ingredients:

- 4 large peaches, pitted and peeled
- 1 onion, finely minced
- ¼ cup ketchup
- ¼ cup low-sodium honey barbecue sauce
- 2 tbsp. brown sugar
- 1 tbsp. low sodium soy sauce
- ¼ tsp. low-sodium garlic salt
- ½ tsp. ground ginger
- 2lb boneless pork chops
- 3 tbsp. olive oil

Directions:

1. Puree the peaches with a blender.
2. Mix the peach puree with the onion, ketchup, barbecue sauce, brown sugar, soy sauce, salt, garlic salt, and ginger.
3. Brown the pork chops in a large skillet then transfer to a 6-quart or larger slow cooker.
4. Pour the sauce over the pork chops and cover.
5. Cook for 5 to 6 hs on high.

Nutrition - Per Serv.: Calories: 252, fat 8g, Carbs 18g, protein 26g, fiber 1g, Potassium 710mg, Sodium 325mg

220.   CHICKEN AVOCADO SALAD

Preparation Time: 8 min.   **Cooking Time:** 20 min.   **Servings**: 8

Ingredients:

- 3 avocados - peeled, pitted and diced
- 1-pound grilled skinless, boneless chicken breast, diced
- ½ cup finely chopped red onion
- ½ cup chopped fresh cilantro
- ¼ cup balsamic vinaigrette salad dressing

Directions:

1. Mix together the chicken, avocados, cilantro, and onion in a medium-sized bowl. Pour over the balsamic vinaigrette dressing. Toss lightly to coat all the ingredients.

Nutrition - Per Serving: Calories: 252; Fat: 17.5 g; Carbs: 8.3g; Protein: 17.2 g; Cholesterol: 43 mg; Sodium: 130 mg; Potassium: 368mg

221.   CHICKEN MANGO SALSA SALAD WITH CHIPOTLE LIME VINAIGRETTE

Preparation Time: 30 min.   **Cooking Time:** 30 min.   **Servings**: 6

Ingredients:

- 1 mango - peeled, seeded and diced
- 2 roam (plum) tomatoes, chopped
- 1/2 onion, chopped
- 1 jalapeno pepper, seeded and chopped - or to taste
- 1/4cupcilantro leaves, chopped
- 1 lime, juiced
- 1/2cupolive oil
- 1/4cuplime juice
- 1/4cupwhite sugar
- 1/2 tsp. Ground chipotle chile powder
- 1/2 tsp. Ground cumin
- 1/4 tsp. Garlic powder
- 1 (10 ounce) bag baby spinach leaves
- 1cupbroccoli coleslaw mix
- 1cupdiced cooked chicken
- 3 tbsp. Diced red bell pepper
- 3 tbsp. Diced green bell pepper
- 2 tbsp. Diced yellow bell pepper
- 2 tbsp. Dried cranberries
- 2 tbsp. Chopped pecans
- 2 tbsp. Crumbled blue cheese

Directions:

1. In a big bowl, combine the jalapeno pepper, juiced lime, mango, cilantro, tomatoes, and onion. Set the mixture aside. In a separate bowl, whisk together the garlic powder, olive oil, cumin, a quarters lime juice, chipotle, and sugar. Set the mixture aside.
2. In another big bowl, toss together the cranberries, spinach, broccoli coleslaw mix, pecans, chicken, and yellow, green and red bell peppers.
3. Top with blue cheese and mango salsa. Make sure they're spread all over.
4. Drizzle the dressing over salad. Toss to serve.

Nutrition - Per Serving: Calories: 317; Fat: 22.3 g; Carbs: 25g; Protein: 7.6 g; Cholesterol: 14 mg; Sodium: 110 mg; Potassium:499 mg

222.   CHICKEN SALAD BALSAMIC

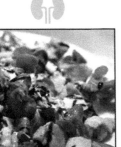

Preparation Time: 15 min.

Cooking Time: 15 min.

Servings: 6

Nutrition - Per Serving:

Calories: 336

Fat: 26.8 g;

Carbs: 6g;

Protein: 19 g

Cholesterol: 55 mg;

Sodium: 58 mg;

Potassium: 267mg

Ingredients:

- 3 cup diced cold, cooked chicken
- 1 cup diced apple
- 1/2 cup diced celery
- 2 green onions, chopped
- 1/2 cup chopped walnuts
- 3 tbsp. Balsamic vinegar
- 5 tbsp. Olive oil
- Salt and pepper to taste

Directions:

1. Toss together the celery, chicken, onion, walnuts, and apple in a big bowl.
2. Whisk the oil together with the vinegar in a small bowl. Pour the dressing over the salad. Then add pepper and salt to taste. Combine the ingredients thoroughly. Leave the mixture for 10-15 min. Toss once more and chill.

223. CHICKEN SALAD WITH APPLES, GRAPES, AND WALNUTS

Preparation Time: 25 min.   **Cooking Time:** 25 min.   **Servings**: 12

Ingredients:

- 4 cooked chicken breasts, shredded
- 2 granny smith apples, cut into small chunks
- 2 cup chopped walnuts, or to taste
- 1/2 red onion, chopped
- 3 stalks celery, chopped
- 3 tbsp. Lemon juice
- ½ cup vanilla yogurt
- 5 tbsp., Creamy salad dressing (such as miracle whip®)
- 5 tbsp. Mayonnaise
- 25 seedless red grapes, halved

Directions:

1. In a big bowl, toss together the shredded chicken, lemon juice, apple chunks, celery, red onion, and walnuts.
2. Get another bowl and whisk together the dressing, vanilla yogurt, and mayonnaise. Pour over the chicken mixture. Toss to coat. Fold the grapes carefully into the salad.

Nutrition - Per Serving: Calories:307; Fat: 22.7g; Carbs: 10.8g; Protein: 17.3 g; Cholesterol: 41 mg; Sodium: 128 mg; Potassium: 818mg

224. CHICKEN STRAWBERRY SPINACH SALAD WITH GINGER-LIME DRESSING

Preparation Time: 10 min.   **Cooking Time:** 30 min.   **Servings**: 2

Ingredients:

- 2 tsp., corn oil
- 1 skinless, boneless chicken breast half - cut into bite-size pieces
- 1/2 tsp., garlic powder
- 1/2 tbsp., mayonnaise
- 1/2 lime, juiced
- 1/2 tsp., ground ginger
- 2 tsp., milk

- 2 cup fresh spinach, stems removed
- 4 fresh strawberries, sliced
- 1/2 tbsp., slivered almonds
- Freshly ground black pepper to taste

Directions:

1. In a skillet, heat oil over medium heat. Add the chicken breast and garlic powder. Cook the chicken for 10 min. per side. When the juices run clear, remove from heat and set aside.
2. Combine the lime juice, milk, mayonnaise, and ginger in a bowl.
3. Place the spinach on serving dishes. Top with strawberries and chicken. Then sprinkle with almonds. Drizzle the salad with the dressing. Add pepper and serve.

Nutrition - Per Serving: Calories: 242 Total fat: 17.3 g; Carbs: 7.5g; Protein: 15.8 g; Cholesterol: 40 mg; Sodium: 117 mg; Potassium: 58mg

225. ASIAN CHICKEN SATAY

Preparation Time: 15 min.   **Cooking Time:** 10 min.   **Servings**: 6

Ingredients:

- 2 limes, Juice
- 2 tbsp., Brown sugar
- 1 tbsp., Minced garlic
- 2 tsp., Ground cumin
- 12 Boneless, skinless chicken breast - cut into strips

Directions:

1. In a bowl, stir together the cumin, garlic, brown sugar, and lime juice. Add the chicken strips to the bowl and marinate in the refrigerator for 1 h.
2. Heat the barbecue to medium-high.
3. Remove the chicken from the marinade and thread each strip onto wooden skewers that have been soaked in the water.
4. Grill the chicken for about 4 min. per side or until the meat is cooked through but still juicy.

Nutrition - Per Serving: Calories: 78; Carbs: 4g; Phosphorus: 116mg; Potassium: 108mg; Sodium: 100mg; Protein: 12g; Potassium: 25mg

226. ZUCCHINI AND TURKEY BURGER WITH JALAPENO PEPPERS

Preparation Time: 15 min.   **Cooking Time:** 10 min.   **Servings**: 4

Ingredients:

- 1 pound, Turkey meat (ground)
- 1 cup, Zucchini (shredded)
- ½ cup, Onion (minced)
- 1 Jalapeño pepper (seeded and minced)
- 1 Egg
- 1 tsp., Extra-spicy blend
- Fresh poblano peppers (seeded and sliced in half lengthwise)
- 1 tsp., Mustard

Directions:

1. Start by taking a mixing bowl and adding turkey meat, zucchini, onion, jalapeño pepper, egg, and extra-spicy blend. Mix well to combine.
2. Divide the mixture into 4 equal portions. Form burger patties out of the same.
3. Prepare an electric griddle or an outdoor grill. Place the burger patties on the grill and cook until the top is blistered and tender. Place the sliced poblano peppers on the grill alongside the patties. Grilling the patties should take about 5 min. on each side.
4. Once done, place the patties onto the buns and top them with grilled peppers.

Nutrition - Per Serving: Protein: 25 g; Carbs: 5 g; Fat: 10 g; Cholesterol: 125 mg; Sodium: 128 mg; Potassium: 475 mg; Phosphorus: 280 mg; Calcium: 43 mg; Fiber: 1.6 g

227.   GNOCCHI AND CHICKEN DUMPLINGS

Preparation Time: 10 min.   **Cooking Time:** 40 min.   **Servings**: 10

Ingredients:

- 2 pounds, Chicken breast
- 1 pound, Gnocchi
- ¼ cup, Light olive oil
- 1 tbsp., Better Than Bouillon® Chicken Base
- 6 cups, Chicken stock (reduced sodium)
- ½ cup, Fresh celery (diced finely)

- ½ cup, Fresh onions (diced finely)
- ½ cup, Fresh carrots (diced finely)
- ¼ cup, Fresh parsley (chopped)
- 1 tsp., Black pepper
- 1 tsp., Italian seasoning

Directions:

1. Start by placing the stock over a high flame. Add in the oil and let it heat through.
2. Add the chicken to the hot oil and shallow fry until all sides turn golden brown.
3. Toss in the carrots, onions, and celery and cook for about 5 min. Pour in the chicken stock and let it cool on a high flame for about 30 min.
4. Reduce the flame and add in the chicken bouillon, Italian seasoning, and black pepper. Stir well.
5. Toss in the store-bought gnocchi and let it cook for about 15 min. Keep stirring.
6. Once done, transfer into a serving bowl. Add parsley and serve hot!

Nutrition - Per Serving: Protein: 28 g; Carbs: 38 g; Fat: 10 g; Cholesterol: 58 mg; Sodium: 121 mg; Potassium: 485 mg; Calcium: 38 mg; Fiber: 2 g

CHAPTER 11. SOUP RECIPES

228. PESTO GREEN VEGETABLE SOUP

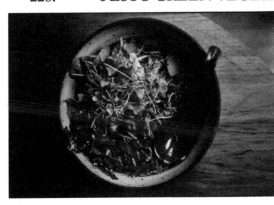

Preparation Time: 10 min.

Cooking Time: 15 min.

Servings: 1

Nutrition - Per Serving: Calories: 170 Fat: 13g

Carbs: 8g

Protein: 3g

Sodium: 333mg

Phosphorus: 42mg

Potassium: 200mg

Ingredients:

- 2 tsp. olive oil
- 1 sliced leek, white and light green
- 2 celery stalks, diced
- 1 tsp. minced garlic
- 2 cups sodium-free chicken stock
- 1 cup chopped snow peas
- 1 cup shredded spinach
- 1 tbsp. chopped fresh thyme
- Juice and zest of ½ lemon
- ¼ tsp. freshly ground black pepper
- 1 tbsp. Basil Pesto

Directions:

1. Add olive oil in a large saucepan.
2. Add the leek, celery, and garlic, and sauté until tender, about 3 min. Stir in the stock and bring to a boil. Stir in the snow peas, spinach, and thyme, and simmer for about 5 min.
3. Remove the pan from the heat, and stir in the lemon juice, lemon zest, pepper, and pesto.
4. Serve immediately.

229. EASY LOW-SODIUM CHICKEN BROTH

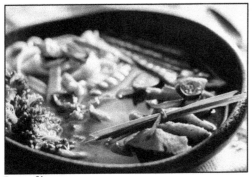

Preparation Time: 10 min.

Cooking Time: 4 hs

Servings: 1

Nutrition - Per Serving: Calories: 32 Carbs: 8g

Protein: 1g

Sodium: 57mg

Potassium: 187mg

Phosphorus: 50mg

Ingredients:

- 2 pounds skinless whole chicken, cut into pieces
- 4 garlic cloves, lightly crushed
- 2 celery stalks, with greens, roughly chopped
- 2 carrots, roughly chopped
- 1 sweet onion, cut into quarters
- 10 peppercorns
- 4 fresh thyme sprigs
- 2 bay leaves
- Water

Directions:

1. In a large stockpot, place the chicken, garlic, celery, carrots, onion, peppercorns, thyme, and bay leaves, and cover with water by about 3 inches. Let the water boil over high heat. Simmer for about 4 hs in low heat.
2. Skim off any foam on top of the stock and pour the stock through a fine-mesh sieve.
3. Pick off all the usable chicken meat for another recipe, discard the bones and other solids, and allow the stock to cool for about 30 min. before transferring it to sealable containers.
4. You can put the stock in the refrigerator for 1 week or up to 2 months in the freezer.

230. CREAM OF SPINACH SOUP

Preparation Time: 15 min.   **Cooking Time:** 30 min.   **Servings**: 4

Ingredients:

- 1 tbsp. olive oil
- ½ sweet onion, chopped
- 2 tsp. minced garlic
- 4 cups fresh spinach
- ¼ cup chopped fresh parsley
- 3 cups of water
- ¼ cup heavy (whipping) cream
- 1 tbsp. freshly squeezed lemon juice
- Freshly ground black pepper

Directions:

1. On a heated olive oil, sauté the onion and garlic in a large saucepan for 3 min.
2. Add the spinach and parsley, and sauté for 5 min.
3. Stir in the water, bring to a boil, then reduce the heat to low. Simmer the soup until the vegetables are tender, about 20 min.
4. Let it cool for 5 min. Then, along with the heavy cream, purée the soup in batches in a food processor (or a blender or a handheld immersion blender).
5. Return the soup to the pot and cook through on low heat. Add the lemon juice, season with pepper, and stir to combine. Serve hot.

Nutrition - Per Serving: Calories: 141; Fat: 14g; Carbs: 3g; Protein: 2g; Sodium: 36mg; Phosphorus: 38mg: Potassium: 200mg

231. VEGETABLE MINESTRONE

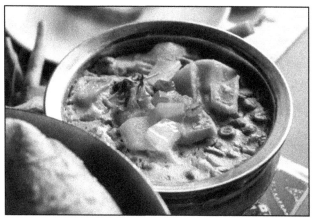

Preparation Time: 20 min.

Cooking Time: 20 min.

Servings: 6

Nutrition - Per Serving: Calories: 100

Fat: 3g;

Carbs: 6g

Protein: 4g

Sodium: 195mg

Phosphorus: 70mg

Potassium: 200mg

Ingredients:

- 1 tsp. olive oil
- ½ sweet onion, chopped
- 1 celery stalk, diced
- 1 tsp. minced garlic
- 2 cups sodium-free chicken stock
- 2 medium tomatoes, chopped
- 1 zucchini, diced
- ½ cup shredded stemmed kale

- Freshly ground black pepper
- 1-ounce grated Parmesan cheese

Directions:

1. Prepare a large saucepan over medium-high heat.
2. Add the onion, celery, and garlic. Sauté until softened, about 5 min.
3. Stir in the stock, tomatoes, and zucchini, and bring to a boil. Let it simmer for 15 min.
4. Stir in the kale and season with pepper.
5. Garnish with the parmesan cheese and serve.

232. VIBRANT CARROT SOUP

Preparation Time: 15 min.   **Cooking Time:** 25 min.   **Servings:** 4

Ingredients:

- 1 tbsp. olive oil
- ½ sweet onion, chopped
- 2 tsp. grated peeled fresh ginger
- 1 tsp. minced fresh garlic
- 4 cups of water
- 3 carrots, chopped
- 1 tsp. ground turmeric
- ½ cup of coconut milk
- 1 tbsp. chopped fresh cilantro

Directions:

1. Heat the olive oil in a saucepan. Sauté the onion, ginger, and garlic until softened.
2. Stir in the water, carrots, and turmeric. Bring the soup to a boil, reduce the heat to low, and simmer until the carrots are tender about 20 min.
3. Transfer the soup in batches to a food processor (or blender) and process with the coconut milk until the soup is smooth.
4. Reheat the soup in a pan.
5. Serve topped with the cilantro.

Nutrition - Per Serving: Calories: 113; Fat: 10g; Protein: 1g; Carbs: 7g; Sodium: 30 mg; Phosphorus: 50 mg; Potassium: 200 mg

233. SIMPLE CABBAGE SOUP

Preparation Time: 20 min.   **Cooking Time:** 35 min.   **Servings:** 8

Ingredients:

- 1 tbsp. olive oil
- ½ sweet onion, chopped
- 2 tsp. minced garlic
- 6 cups of water
- 1 cup sodium-free chicken stock
- ½ head green cabbage, shredded
- 2 carrots, diced
- 2 medium tomatoes, diced
- Freshly ground black pepper
- 2 tbsp. chopped fresh thyme

Directions:

1. Prepare olive oil in a large saucepan over medium-high heat.
2. Sauté the onion and garlic until softened.
3. Add water, chicken stock, cabbage, carrots, and tomatoes. Let it bring it to a boil.
4. In medium-low heat, simmer the vegetables for 30 min. or until tender.
5. Season the soup with black pepper. Serve hot, topped with the thyme.

Nutrition - Per Serving: Calories: 62; Fat: 2g; Carbs: 6g; Protein: 2g; Sodium: 61mg; Phosphorus: 32mg; Potassium: 200mg

234. MUSHROOM MOCK MISO SOUP

Preparation Time: 10 min. **Cooking Time:** 35 min. **Servings**: 6

Ingredients:

- 6 cups water, divided
- 2 ounces dried mixed mushrooms
- ¼ cup of seasoned rice vinegar
- 1 tsp. low-sodium soy sauce
- 1 tbsp. grated peeled fresh ginger
- 1 cup julienned snow peas
- ½ cup grated carrot
- 2 scallions, green and white parts, chopped

Directions:

1. Prepare 2 cups of water in a small saucepan over high heat and bring to a boil.
2. Place the dried mushrooms in a medium bowl and pour the boiling water over them. Let the mushrooms reconstitute for 30 min., then remove them from the water and slice them thinly.
3. Transfer the mushroom water, the remaining 4 cups of water, vinegar, soy sauce, ginger to a large saucepan, and place over medium-high heat.
4. Bring to a boil, then put mushrooms, snow peas, and carrot. Reduce the heat to low, and simmer for 5 min. Serve hot, topped with the scallions.

Nutrition - Per Serving: Calories: 56; Fat: 0g; Carbs: 9g; Protein: 2g; Sodium: 118mg; Phosphorus: 43mg; Potassium: 198mg

235. FENNEL CAULIFLOWER SOUP

Preparation Time: 20 min. **Cooking Time:** 30 min. **Servings**: 1

Ingredients:

- 1 tsp. olive oil
- 1 small, sweet onion, chopped
- 2 tsp. minced garlic
- ½ small head cauliflower, cut into small florets
- 2 cups chopped fresh fennel
- 4 cups of water
- 2 tsp. chopped fresh thyme
- ¼ cup heavy (whipping) cream

Directions:

1. Prepare a saucepan and heat the olive oil.
2. Put onion and garlic. Sauté until softened, about 3 min.
3. Add the cauliflower, fennel, and water. Let it boil, then reduce the heat to medium-low and simmer until the cauliflower is tender, about 20 min.
4. In batches, pour the soup into a food processor (or blender), and purée until smooth and creamy.
5. Return the soup to the pan. Stir in the thyme and cream—heat on medium-low until warmed through, about 5 min. Serve.

Nutrition: Calories: 105; Fat: 8g; Carbs: 5g; Protein: 1g; Sodium: 30mg; Phosphorus: 41mg; Potassium: 200mg

236. CHICKEN ALPHABET SOUP

Preparation Time: 15 min. **Cooking Time:** 35 min. **Servings**: 6

Ingredients:

- 1 tbsp. olive oil
- ½ sweet onion, diced
- 2 tsp. minced garlic
- 4 cups of water
- 1½ cups chopped cooked chicken breast
- 1 cup sodium-free chicken stock
- 2 celery stalks, chopped
- 1 carrot, peeled and diced
- ½ cup dried alphabet noodles
- Freshly ground black pepper
- 2 tbsp. chopped fresh parsley

Directions:

1. Put olive oil in a large saucepan with medium-high heat.
2. Add the onion and garlic. Cook until softened, about 3 min.
3. Add the water, chicken, chicken stock, celery, and carrot. Bring to a boil, then reduce the heat to medium-low and simmer until the vegetables are tender-crisp about 15 min.
4. Add the noodles, stir, and simmer the soup until the noodles are tender about 15 min.
5. Season with pepper. Serve hot with topped parsley.

Nutrition - Per Serving: Calories: 132; Fat: 3g; Carbs: 10g; Protein: 13g; Sodium: 95mg; Phosphorus: 116mg; Potassium: 200mg

237.   MEATBALL SOUP

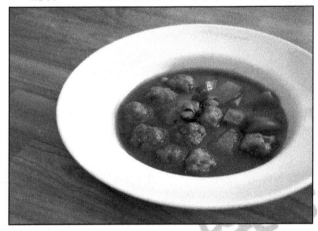

Preparation Time: 20 min.

Cooking Time: 40 min.

Servings: 6

Nutrition - Per Serving:

Calories: 106

Fat: 3g

Carbs: 4g

Protein: 9g

Sodium: 53mg

Phosphorus: 92mg

Potassium: 200mg

Ingredients:

- ½ pound lean ground beef
- 2 tbsp. breadcrumbs
- 1 tbsp. chopped fresh parsley
- 1 tsp. minced garlic
- 1 tsp. olive oil
- ½ sweet onion, chopped
- 5 cups of water
- 2 tomatoes, chopped
- 2 celery stalks with the greens, chopped
- 1 carrot, diced
- Freshly ground black pepper

Directions:

1. Mix the ground beef, breadcrumbs, parsley, and garlic in a large bowl. Roll the meat mixture into small (1-inch) meatballs.
2. Add the onion in a large saucepan, and sauté until softened, about 3 min.
3. Add the water, tomatoes, celery, and carrot, and bring to a boil. Add the meatballs, reduce the heat to medium-low, and simmer until the vegetables are tender and the meatballs are cooked through about 35 min.
4. Season the soup with pepper and serve hot.

238.   VEGETABLE STEW

Preparation Time: 15 min.   **Cooking Time:** 15 min.   **Servings**: 8

Ingredients:

- 1 tsp. olive oil
- 1 sweet onion, chopped
- 1 tsp. minced garlic
- 2 zucchinis, chopped
- 1 red bell pepper, diced
- 2 carrots, chopped

- 2 cups low-sodium vegetable stock
- 2 large tomatoes, chopped
- 2 cups broccoli florets
- 1 tsp. ground coriander
- ½ tsp. ground cumin
- Pinch cayenne pepper
- Freshly ground black pepper
- 2 tbsp. chopped fresh cilantro

Directions:

1. Cook garlic and onion in a saucepan until softened.
2. Put zucchini, bell pepper, and carrots, and sauté for 5 min.
3. Mix vegetable stock, tomatoes, broccoli, coriander, cumin, and cayenne pepper.
4. Let it boil and simmer to medium-low until the vegetables are tender, often stirring about 5 min.
5. Add pepper and serve hot, topped with the cilantro.

Nutrition: Calories: 45; Fat: 1g; Carbs: 5g; Protein: 1g; Sodium: 194mg; Phosphorus: 21mg; Potassium: 184mg

239.   SAUSAGE & EGG SOUP

Preparation Time: 15 min.   **Cooking Time:** 30 min.   **Servings**: 4

Ingredients:

- 1/2 lb. ground beef
- Black pepper
- 1/2 tsp. ground sage
- 1/2 tsp. garlic powder
- 1/2 tsp. dried basil
- 4 slices bread (one day old), cubed
- 2 tbsp. olive oil
- 1 tbsp. herb seasoning blend
- 2 garlic cloves, minced
- 3 cups low-sodium chicken broth
- 1 cup of water
- 4 tbsp. fresh parsley
- 4 eggs
- 2 tbsp. Parmesan cheese, grated

Directions:

1. Preheat your oven to 375 F.
2. Mix the first five ingredients to make the sausage—Toss bread cubes in oil and seasoning blend. Bake in the oven for 8 min. Set aside.
3. Cook the sausage in a pan over medium heat.
4. Cook the garlic in the sausage drippings for 2 min.
5. Stir in the broth, water, and parsley and let it boil. Simmer for 10 min.
6. Pour into serving bowls and top with baked bread, egg, and sausage.

Nutrition - Per Serving: Calories: 196; Fat: 11g; Carbs: 17g; Protein: 7g; Sodium: 148mg; Potassium: 537mg; Phosphorus: 125mg

240.   SEAFOOD CHOWDER WITH CORN

Preparation Time: 15 min.   **Cooking Time:** 20 min.   **Servings**: 10

Ingredients:

- 1 tbsp. butter (unsalted)
- 1 cup onion, chopped
- ½ cup red bell pepper, chopped
- ½ cup green bell pepper, chopped
- ¼ cup celery, chopped
- 1 tbsp. all-purpose white flour
- 14 oz. low-sodium chicken broth
- 2 cups non-dairy creamer
- 6 oz. almond milk
- 10 oz. crab flakes
- 2 cups corn kernels
- ½ tsp. paprika
- Black pepper to taste

Directions:

1. Melt the butter in a pan. Cook the onion, bell peppers, and celery for 4 min. Stir in the flour and cook for 2 min.
2. Add the broth and bring to a boil.
3. Add the rest of the ingredients.
4. Stir occasionally and cook for 5 min.

Nutrition - Per Serving: Calories: 156; Fat: 11g; Carbs: 17g; Protein: 7g; Sodium: 128mg; Potassium: 527mg; Phosphorus: 125mg

241.   LAMB STEW

Preparation Time: 30 min.   **Cooking Time:** 1 h 40 min.   **Servings**: 6

Ingredients:
- 1 lb. boneless lamb shoulder, trimmed and cubes
- Black pepper to taste
- 1/4 cup all-purpose flour
- 1 tbsp. olive oil
- 1 onion, chopped
- 3 garlic cloves, chopped
- 1/2 cup tomato sauce
- 2 cups low-sodium beef broth
- 1 tsp. dried thyme
- 2 parsnips, sliced
- 2 carrots, sliced
- 1 cup frozen peas

Directions:
1. Season the lamb with pepper. Coat it evenly with flour. Pour oil into a pot over medium heat. Cook the lamb and then set aside.
2. Add onion to the pot. Cook for 2 min.
3. Add garlic and sauté for 30 seconds.
4. Pour in the broth to deglaze the pot.
5. Add the tomato sauce and thyme.
6. Put the lamb back in the pot.
7. Let it boil and then simmer for 1 h.
8. Add parsnips and carrots—Cook for 30 min.
9. Put green peas and cook for 5 min.

Nutrition - Per Serving: Calories: 156; Fat: 11g; Carbs: 17g; Protein: 7g; Sodium: 148mg; Potassium: 567mg; Phosphorus: 115mg

242.   SPRING VEGGIE SOUP

Preparation Time: 20 min.   **Cooking Time:** 45 min.   **Servings**: 5

Ingredients:
- 2 tbsp. olive oil
- 1/2 cup onion, diced
- 1/2 cup mushrooms, sliced
- 1/8 cup celery, chopped
- 1 tomato, diced
- 1/2 cup carrots, diced
- 1 cup green beans, trimmed
- 1/2 cup frozen corn
- 1 tsp. garlic powder
- 1 tsp. dried oregano leaves
- 4 cups low-sodium vegetable broth

Directions:
1. In a pot, pour the olive oil and cook the onion and celery for 2 min.
2. Add the rest of the ingredients.
3. Bring to a boil.
4. Reduce heat and simmer for 45 min.

Nutrition - Per Serving: Calories: 136; Fat: 11g; Carbs: 17g; Protein: 7g; Sodium: 138mg; Potassium: 527mg; Phosphorus: 125mg

243.   TACO SOUP

Preparation Time: 30 min.   **Cooking Time:** 7 hs   **Servings**: 10

Ingredients:
- 1 lb. chicken breast (boneless, skinless)
- 15 oz. canned red kidney beans
- 15 oz. low-sodium white corn, rinsed and drained

- 15 oz. canned yellow hominy, rinsed and drained
- 1 cup canned tomatoes with green chilies, diced
- 1/2 cup onion, chopped
- 1/2 cup green bell peppers, chopped
- 1 clove garlic, chopped
- 1 jalapeno, chopped
- 1 tbsp. low-sodium taco seasoning
- 2 cups low-sodium chicken broth

Directions:

1. Put the chicken in the slow cooker.
2. Top with the rest of the ingredients. Cook on high for 1 h.
3. Cook in low for 6 hs.
4. Shred chicken and serve with the soup.

Nutrition - Per Serving: Calories: 86; Fat: 18g; Carbs: 17g; Protein: 7g; Sodium: 248mg; Potassium: 517mg; Phosphorus: 125mg

244. CURRIED CARROT AND BEET SOUP

Preparation Time: 10 min.   **Cooking Time:** 50 min.   **Servings**: 4

Ingredients:

- 1 large red beet
- 5 carrots, chopped
- 1 tbsp. curry powder
- 3 cups Homemade Rice Milk or unsweetened store-bought rice milk
- Freshly ground black pepper
- Yogurt, for serving

Directions:

1. Preheat the oven to 400°F.
2. Cover beet in aluminum foil and roast for 45 min., until the vegetable is tender when pierced with a fork. Remove from the oven and let cool. In a saucepan, add the carrots and cover with water. Bring to a boil, reduce the heat, and simmer for 10 min. until tender.
3. Transfer the carrots and beet to a food processor and process until smooth. Add the curry powder and rice milk. Season it with pepper. Serve topped with a dollop of yogurt.

Nutrition - Per Serving: Calories: 186; Fat: 11g; Carbs: 17g; Protein: 7g; Sodium: 248mg; Potassium: 357mg; Phosphorus: 225mg

245. ASPARAGUS LEMON SOUP

Preparation Time: 10 min.   **Cooking Time:** 25 min.   **Servings**: 4

Ingredients:

- 1-pound asparagus
- 2 tbsp. extra-virgin olive oil
- ½ sweet onion, chopped
- 4 cups low-sodium chicken stock
- ½ cup Homemade Rice Milk or unsweetened store-bought rice milk
- Freshly ground black pepper
- Juice of 1 lemon

Directions:

1. Cut the asparagus tips from the spears and set aside. Heat the olive oil in a small stockpot. Add the onion and cook, frequently stirring for 3 to 5 min., until it softens.
2. Add the stock and asparagus stalks and bring to a boil. Reduce the heat and simmer until the asparagus is tender about 15 min.
3. Put to a blender or food processor and carefully purée until smooth. Return to the pot,

add the asparagus tips, and simmer until tender, about 5 min.

4. Add the rice milk, pepper, and lemon juice, and stir until heated through. Serve.

Nutrition - Per Serving: Calories: 86; Fat: 11g; Carbs: 17g; Protein: 7g; Sodium: 128mg; Potassium: 257mg; Phosphorus: 155mg

246. CAULIFLOWER AND CHIVE SOUP

Preparation Time: 10 min.   **Cooking Time:** 20 min.   **Servings**: 4

Ingredients:

- 2 tbsp. extra-virgin olive oil
- ½ sweet onion, chopped
- 2 garlic cloves, minced
- 2 cups Simple Chicken Broth or low-sodium store-bought chicken stock
- 1 cauliflower head, broken into florets
- Freshly ground black pepper
- 4 tbsp. (¼ cups) finely chopped chives

Directions:

1. Heat the olive oil. Add and cook the onion, frequently stirring, until it softens for 3 to 5 min. Add the garlic and stir until fragrant.
2. Add the broth and cauliflower and bring to a boil. Reduce the heat and simmer until the cauliflower is tender about 15 min.
3. Transfer the soup in batches to a blender or food processor and purée until smooth or use an immersion blender.
4. Return the soup to the pot, and season with pepper. Before serving, top each bowl with 1 tbsp. of chives.

Nutrition - Per Serving: Calories: 156; Fat: 11g; Carbs: 17g; Protein: 7g; Sodium: 248mg; Potassium: 527mg; Phosphorus: 125mg

247. SIMPLE CHICKEN AND RICE SOUP

Preparation Time: 10 min.   **Cooking Time:** 15 min.   **Servings**: 4

Ingredients:

- 1 tbsp. extra-virgin olive oil
- ½ sweet onion, chopped
- 2 celery stalks, chopped
- 2 carrots, chopped
- 8 ounces chicken breast, diced
- 4 cups Simple Chicken Broth or low-sodium store-bought chicken stock
- ¼ tsp. dried thyme leaves
- 1 cup cooked rice
- Juice of 1 lime
- Freshly ground black pepper
- 2 tbsp. chopped parsley leaves, for garnish

Directions:

1. Heat the olive oil over medium-high heat. Add the onion, celery, carrots, and cook, often stirring, for about 5 min., until the onion begins to soften.
2. Add the chicken breast and continue stirring until the meat is just browned but not cooked
through. Add the broth and thyme and bring to a boil.
3. Simmer for 10 min., until the chicken is cooked through and the vegetables are tender.
4. Add the rice and lime juice. Season it with pepper. Serve and garnished with parsley leaves.

Nutrition - Per Serving: Calories: 176; Fat: 11g; Carbs: 17g; Protein: 7g; Sodium: 128mg; Potassium: 357mg; Phosphorus: 225mg

248. TURKEY, WILD RICE, AND MUSHROOM SOUP

Preparation Time: 15 min.   **Cooking Time:** 2-3 hs   **Servings**: 6

Ingredients:

- ½ cup onion, chopped
- ½ cup red bell pepper, chopped
- ½ cup carrots, chopped
- 2 garlic cloves, minced
- 2 cup cooked turkey, shredded
- 5 cup chicken broth (see recipe)
- ½ cup quick-cooking wild rice, uncooked
- 1 tbsp. olive oil
- 1 cup mushrooms, sliced
- 2 bay leaves
- ¼ tsp. Mrs. Dash® Original salt-free herb seasoning blend
- 1 tsp. dried thyme
- ½ tsp. low sodium salt
- ¼ tsp. black pepper

Directions:

1. Cook rice in a saucepan with 1-2 cups of broth. Set aside.
2. Heat the oil in a skillet and sauté the onion, bell pepper, carrots, and garlic until soft. Add to a 4 to 6-quart slow cooker.
3. Add remaining ingredients to the slow cooker except for the rice and mushrooms.
4. Cook for 2-3 hs on low with cover.
5. Put the mushrooms and rice. Cook for another 15 min. Remove the bay leaves and serve

Nutrition - Per Serving: Calories: 136; Fat: 11g; Carbs: 15g; Protein: 5g; Sodium: 128mg; Potassium: 537mg; Phosphorus: 145mg

249.   TURKEY BURGER SOUP

Preparation Time: 10min.   **Cooking Time:** 25 min.   **Servings**: 4

Ingredients:

- 2 tbsp. extra-virgin olive oil
- 1-pound ground turkey breast
- ½ sweet onion, chopped
- 3 garlic cloves, minced
- Freshly ground black pepper
- 1 (16-ounce) can low-sodium diced tomatoes, drained
- 4 cups Simple Chicken Broth or low-sodium store-bought chicken stock
- 1 cup sliced carrots
- 1 cup sliced celery
- 1 tbsp. chopped fresh basil
- 1 tbsp. chopped fresh oregano
- 1 tbsp. chopped fresh thyme

Directions:

1. Prepare the olive oil. Add the turkey, onion, and garlic in a medium stockpot.
2. Cook, stirring until the turkey is browned. Season it with pepper.
3. Add the drained tomatoes, broth, carrots, celery, basil, oregano, and thyme.
4. Reduce the heat to low, and simmer for 20 min. Serve.

Nutrition - Per Serving: Calories: 186; Fat: 11g; Carbs: 17g; Protein: 7g; Sodium: 128mg; Potassium: 257mg; Phosphorus: 115mg

CHAPTER 12. EGGS AND DAIRY

250.   CHEESE STUFFED PEPPERS

Preparation Time: 25 min.   **Cooking Time:** 10 min.   **Servings**: 4

Ingredients:

- 4 summer bell peppers, divined and halved
- 2 ounces mozzarella cheese, crumbled
- 2 tbsp. Greek-style yogurt
- 4 ounces cream cheese
- 1 clove garlic, minced

Directions:

1. Boil the peppers until they are just tender.
2. Thoroughly combine the cheese, yogurt, and garlic. Stuff your peppers with this filling. Place the stuffed peppers in a foil-lined baking dish.
3. Bake in the preheated oven at 365 F for about 10 min. Bon appétit!

Nutrition - Per Serving: Calories: 140; Fat: 9g; Carbs: 6g; Protein: 7g; Fiber: 0.9g; Sodium: 469mg; Potassium: 37mg

251.   ITALIAN ZUCCHINI SANDWICHES

Preparation Time: 25 min.   **Cooking Time:** 5 min.   **Servings**: 4

Ingredients:

- 4 thin zucchini slices, cut lengthwise
- 2 eggs
- 4 slices Sopressata
- 2 slices provolone cheese
- 1 red bell pepper, sliced thinly

Directions:

1. Dissolve 1 tbsp. of butter in a frying pan over medium-high flame. Then, fry the eggs for about 5 min.
2. Place one zucchini slice on each plate. Add the cheese, Sopressata, and peppers on top; season with salt and black pepper to taste.
3. Add fried eggs and top with the remaining zucchini slices. Bon appétit!

Nutrition: Calories: 240; Fat: 9g; Carbs: 6g; Protein: 7g; Fiber: 0.9g; Sodium: 604mg; Potassium: 285mg

252.   CREAMY DILLED EGG SALAD

Preparation Time: 20 min.   **Cooking Time:** 11 min.   **Servings**: 3

Ingredients:

- 4 eggs, peeled and chopped
- 1 scallion, chopped
- 1 tbsp. fresh dill minced
- 1 tsp. Dijon mustard
- 4 tbsp. mayonnaise

Directions:

1. Add the eggs and water to a saucepan and bring to a boil; remove from heat. Allow the eggs to sit, covered, for about 11 min.
2. Peel and rinse the eggs under running water. Then, chop the eggs and transfer them to a nice salad bowl; stir in the scallions, dill, mustard, and mayonnaise.
3. Taste and season with salt and pepper. Enjoy!

Nutrition: Calories: 220; Fat: 7g; Carbs: 6g; Protein: 5g; Fiber: 0.9g; Sodium: 241mg; Potassium: 99mg

253.   EGGS WITH GOAT CHEESE

Preparation Time: 10 min.   **Cooking Time:** 10 min.   **Servings**: 2

Ingredients:

- 4 eggs, whisked
- 2 tsp. ghee, room temperature
- 1 tsp. paprika
- Sea salt and ground black pepper, to taste
- 4 tbsp. goat cheese

Directions:

1. In a frying pan, melt the ghee over a moderate heat. Then, cook the eggs, covered, for about 4 min.
2. Stir in goat cheese, paprika, salt, and black pepper; continue to cook for 2 to 3 min. more or until cooked through.
3. Taste and adjust seasonings. Enjoy!

Nutrition - Per Serving: Calories: 210; Fat: 9g; Carbs: 4g; Protein: 7g; Fiber: 0.9g; Sodium: 176mg; Potassium: 146mg

---

254.   Dukkah Frittata with Cheese

Preparation Time: 30 min.   **Cooking Time:** 25 min.   **Servings**: 3

Ingredients:

- 3 tbsp. milk
- 1 tbsp. Dukkha spice mix
- 5 eggs
- 2 tbsp. olive oil
- 1 cup cheddar cheese, shredded

Directions:

1. Preheat your oven to 360 F. Whisk the milk, spices mix and eggs until well mixed.
2. Grease the bottom of a small-sized baking pan with olive oil. Spoon the egg mixture into the pan and top with cheese.
3. Bake in the preheated oven for about 25 min. until the eggs are set but the center jiggles just a bit. Bon appétit!

Nutrition: Calories: 320; Fat: 11g; Carbs: 6g; Protein: 9g; Fiber: 0.9g; Sodium: 344mg; Potassium: 144mg

255.   CLASSIC ITALIAN OMELET

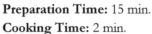

Preparation Time: 15 min.

Cooking Time: 2 min.

Servings: 3

Nutrition - Per Serving: Calories: 308

Fat: 12g

Carbs: 6g

Protein: 10g

Fiber: 0.9g

Sodium: 1152mg

Potassium: 280mg

Ingredients:

- 3 ounces bacon, diced
- 1 Italian pepper, chopped
- 6 eggs, whisked
- 1 tsp. Italian seasoning blend
- 1/2 cup goat cheese, shredded

Directions:

1. Over a medium-high heat, warm the frying pan. Now, fry the bacon until crisp or 3 to 4 min.; set aside.
2. Stir in Italian pepper and continue to sauté for 2 min. more or until just tender and fragrant. Pour the eggs into the pan.
3. Sprinkle with the Italian seasoning blend; add the salt and black pepper to taste and cook until the eggs are ser. Top with the reserved bacon and goat cheese.
4. Slide your omelet onto serving plates and serve. Bon appétit!

256.   EGG SALAD WITH ANCHOVIES

Preparation Time: 15 min.   **Cooking Time:** 10 min.   **Servings**: 3

Ingredients:

- 3 ounces anchovies, flaked
- 5 eggs
- 2 tbsp. mayonnaise
- 1 tsp. Dijon mustard
- 2 tbsp. Ricotta cheese

Directions:

1. Add the eggs and water to a saucepan and bring to a boil; remove from heat. Allow the eggs to sit, covered, for about 11 min.
2. Then, peel the eggs and rinse them under running water. Then, transfer chopped eggs to a salad bowl. Add in the remaining ingredients, gently stir to combine and enjoy!

Nutrition - Per Serving: Calories: 240; Fat: 9g; Carbs: 6g; Protein: 7g; Fiber: 0.9g; Sodium: 1244mg; Potassium: 269mg

257.   CLASSIC MUFFINS

Preparation Time: 20 min.   **Cooking Time:** 16 min.   **Servings**: 4

Ingredients:

- 4 ounces cheddar cheese, shredded
- 6 tbsp. almond flour
- 2 tbsp. flaxseed meal
- 4 eggs
- 1/4 tsp. baking soda

Directions:

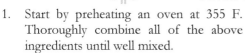

1. Start by preheating an oven at 355 F. Thoroughly combine all of the above ingredients until well mixed.

2. Coat a muffin pan with cupcake liners. Spoon the batter into the muffin pan. Bake in the preheated oven for 16 min.

3. Place on a wire rack for 10 min. before unmolding and serving. Enjoy!

Nutrition - Per Serving: Calories: 213; Fat: 9g; Carbs: 6g; Protein: 7g; Fiber: 0.9g; Sodium: 318mg; Potassium: 115mg

258. AUTHENTIC SPANISH MIGAS

Preparation Time: 15 min.   **Cooking Time:** 10 min.   **Servings**: 3

Ingredients:

- 6 eggs
- 6 lettuce leaves
- 1 white onion, chopped
- 1 tomato, chopped
- 1 Spanish pepper, chopped

Directions:

1. Melt 1 tbsp. of butter in a cast-iron skillet over medium-high flame. Sauté the onion for about 4 min., stirring continuously to ensure even cooking.

2. Stir in the peppers and continue to sauté an additional 3 to 4 min. Whisk in the eggs. Continue to cook until the eggs are set.

3. Divide the egg mixture between lettuce leaves, top with tomatoes. Season with salt and black pepper and serve. Devour!

Nutrition - Per Serving: Calories: 256; Fat: 8g; Carbs: 6g; Protein: 10g; Fiber: 0.9g; Sodium: 165mg; Potassium: 235mg

259. DOUBLE CHEESE FONDUE

Preparation Time: 10 min.   **Cooking Time:** 0 min.   **Servings**: 8

Ingredients:

- 4 ounces Ricotta cheese
- 1 cup double cream
- Cayenne pepper, to taste
- 8 ounces Swiss cheese, shredded
- 4 tbsp.
- Greek-style yogurt

Directions:

1. Warm Ricotta cheese and double cream and in a saucepan over medium-low flame.

2. Remove from the heat. Fold in cayenne pepper, Swiss cheese, and Greek-style yogurt. Stir until everything is well combined.

3. Bon appétit!

Nutrition: Calories: 230; Fat: 9g; Carbs: 6g; Protein: 7g; Fiber: 0.9g; Sodium: 90mg; Potassium: 51mg

260. SAVORY ROLLS WITH BACON AND CHEESE

Preparation Time: 30 min.   **Cooking Time:** 14 min.   **Servings**: 8

Ingredients:

- 1/2 cup goat cheese, crumbled
- 1/2 cup cream cheese
- 8 eggs
- 6 ounces bacon, diced
- 1/2 cup marinara sauce

Directions:

1. In a coated skillet, fry the bacon over the highest heat until crisp; set aside.
2. Whisk the cream cheese and eggs until foamy. Add in the fried bacon along with salt and black pepper; whisk to combine well.
3. Spoon the mixture into greased muffin cups. Top each muffin with goat cheese. Bake in the heated oven at 355 F for about 14 min. or until golden on the top. Serve with marinara sauce and enjoy!

Nutrition: Calories: 308; Fat: 9g; Carbs: 9g; Protein: 12g; Fiber: 0.9g; Sodium: 758mg; Potassium: 259mg

261.   BROCCOLI CHEESE PIE

Preparation Time: 30 min.   **Cooking Time:** 20 min.   **Servings**: 4

Ingredients:

- 6 eggs
- 1 red onion, sliced
- 6 tbsp. Greek yogurt
- 2 cups broccoli florets
- 1/2 cup cheddar cheese, shredded

Directions:

1. Heat 2 tsp. of olive oil in an oven-safe skillet over medium-high heat. Sweat red onion and broccoli until they have softened or about 4 min. Season with salt and black pepper.
2. In a mixing bowl, whisk Greek yogurt and eggs until well mixed. Scrape the mixture into the pan.
3. Bake at 365 F for 15 to 20 min. or until a toothpick inserted into a muffin comes out dry and clean.
4. Top with cheddar cheese and bake for 5 to 6 min. more. Bon appétit!

Nutrition: Calories: 140; Fat: 9g; Carbs: 6g; Protein: 7g; Fiber: 0.9g; Sodium: 213mg; Potassium: 357mg

CHAPTER 13. SALAD RECIPES

262.   PEAR & BRIE SALAD

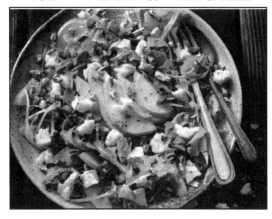

Preparation Time: 5 min.

Cooking Time: 0 min.

Servings: 4

Nutrition - Per Serving: Calories: 54

Protein 1 g

Carbs 12 g

Fat 7 g

Sodium 57mg

Potassium 115 mg

Phosphorus 67 mg

Ingredients:
- 1 tbsp. olive oil
- 1 cup arugula
- ½ lemon
- ½ cup canned pears
- ¼ cucumber
- ¼ cup chopped brie

Directions:
1. Peel and dice the cucumber.
2. Dice the pear.
3. Wash the arugula.
4. Combine salad in a serving bowl and crumble the brie over the top.
5. Whisk the olive oil and lemon juice together.
6. Drizzle over the salad.
7. Season with a little black pepper to taste and serve immediately.

263.   CAESAR SALAD

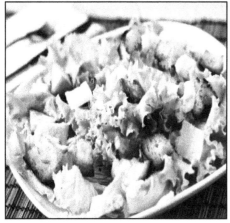

Preparation Time: 5 min.

Cooking Time: 5 min.

Servings: 4

Ingredients:
- 1 head romaine lettuce
- ¼ cup mayonnaise
- 1 tbsp. lemon juice
- 4 anchovy fillets
- 1 tsp. Worcestershire sauce
- Black pepper
- 5 garlic cloves
- 4 tbsp. Parmesan cheese
- 1 tsp. mustard

Directions:
1. In a bowl mix all ingredients and mix well
2. Serve with dressing

Nutrition - Per Serving: Calories: 44; Fat 2.1 g; Sodium 83 mg; Potassium 216 mg; Carbs 4.3 g; Protein 3.2 g; Phosphorus 45.6mg

264. THAI CUCUMBER SALAD

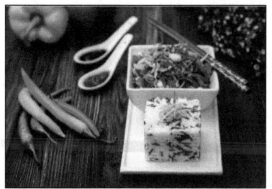

Preparation Time: 5 min.

Cooking Time: 5 min.

Servings: 2

Ingredients:

- ¼ cup chopped peanuts
- ¼ cup white sugar
- ½ cup cilantro
- ¼ cup rice wine vinegar
- 3 cucumbers
- 2 jalapeno peppers

Directions:

1. In a bowl add all ingredients and mix well
2. Serve with dressing

Nutrition - Per Serving: Calories: 20; Fat 0g; Sodium 85mg; Carbs 5g; Protein 1g; Potassium 190.4 mg; Phosphorus 46.8mg

265. BROCCOLI-CAULIFLOWER SALAD

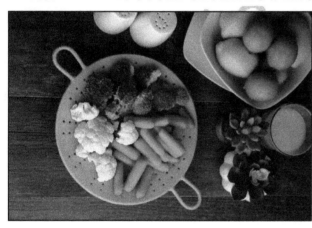

Preparation Time: 5 min.

Cooking Time: 5 min.

Servings: 4

Nutrition - Per Serving:

Calories: 89.8;

Fat 4.5g;

Sodium 51.2mg;

Potassium 257.6mg;

Carbs 11.5g;

Protein 3.0g;

Phosphorus 47 mg

Ingredients:

- 1 tbsp. wine vinegar
- 1 cup cauliflower florets
- ¼ cup white sugar
- 2 cups hard-cooked eggs
- 5 slices bacon
- 1 cup broccoli florets
- 1 cup cheddar cheese
- 1 cup mayonnaise

Directions:

1. In a bowl add all ingredients and mix well
2. Serve with dressing

266. GREEN BEAN AND POTATO SALAD

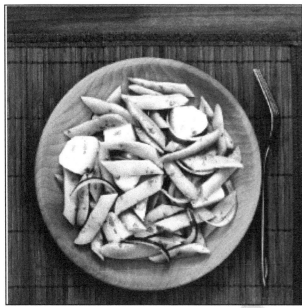

Preparation Time: 5 min.

Cooking Time: 5 min.

Servings: 4

Nutrition - Per Serving: Calories: 153.2

Fat 2.0 g

Carbs 29.0 g

Protein 6.9 g

Sodium 77.6 mg

Potassium 759.0 mg

Phosphorus 49 mg

Ingredients:

- ½ cup basil
- ¼ cup olive oil
- 1 tbsp. mustard
- ¾ lb. green beans
- 1 tbsp. lemon juice
- ½ cup balsamic vinegar
- 1 red onion
- 1 lb. red potatoes
- 1 garlic clove

Directions:

1. Place potatoes in a pot with water and bring to a boil for 15-18 min. or until tender
2. Thrown in green beans after 5-6 min.
3. Drain and cut into cubes
4. In a bowl add all ingredients and mix well
5. Serve with dressing

267. ITALIAN CUCUMBER SALAD

Preparation Time: 5 min.   **Cooking Time:** 0 min.   **Servings**: 2

Ingredients:

- 1/4 cup rice vinegar
- 1/8 tsp. stevia
- 1/2 tsp. olive oil
- 1/8 tsp. black pepper
- 1/2 cucumber, sliced
- 1 cup carrots, sliced
- 2 tbsp. green onion, sliced
- 2 tbsp. red bell pepper, sliced
- 1/2 tsp. Italian seasoning blend

Directions:

1. Put all the salad ingredients into a suitable salad bowl.
2. Toss them well and refrigerate for 1 h.
3. Serve.

Nutrition - Per Serving: Calories: 112; Total Fat 1.6g; Cholesterol 0mg; Protein 2.3g; Sodium 43mg; Phosphorous 198mg; Potassium 529mg

268. GRAPES JICAMA SALAD

Preparation Time: 5 min.   **Cooking Time:** 0 min.   **Servings**: 2

Ingredients:

- 1 jicama, peeled and sliced
- 1 carrot, sliced
- 1/2 medium red onion, sliced
- 1 ¼ cup seedless grapes
- 1/3 cup fresh basil leaves
- 1 tbsp. apple cider vinegar
- 1 ½ tbsp. lemon juice

↳ 1 ½ tbsp. lime juice

Directions:

1. Put all the salad ingredients into a suitable salad bowl.
2. Toss them well and refrigerate for 1 h.
3. Serve.

Nutrition - Per Serving: Calories: 203; Fat 0.7g; Sodium 44mg; Protein 3.7g; Calcium 79mg; Phosphorous 141mg; Potassium 429mg

269.   CUCUMBER COUSCOUS SALAD

Preparation Time: 5 min.   **Cooking Time:** 0 min.   **Servings**: 4

Ingredients:

- 1 cucumber, sliced
- ½ cup red bell pepper, sliced
- ¼ cup sweet onion, sliced
- 2 tbsp. black olives, sliced
- ¼ cup parsley, chopped
- ½ cup couscous, cooked
- 2 tbsp. olive oil
- 2 tbsp. rice vinegar
- 2 tbsp. feta cheese crumbled
- 1 ½ tsp. dried basil
- 1/4 tsp. black pepper

Directions:

1. Put all the salad ingredients into a suitable salad bowl.
2. Toss them well and refrigerate for 1 h.
3. Serve.

Nutrition - Per Serving: Calories: 202; Fat 9.8g; Sodium 258mg; Protein 6.2g; Calcium 80mg; Phosphorous 192mg; Potassium 209mg

270.   CARROT JICAMA SALAD

Preparation Time: 5 min.   **Cooking Time:** 0 min.   **Servings**: 2

Ingredients:

- 2 cup carrots, julienned
- 1 1/2 cups jicama, julienned
- 2 tbsp. lime juice
- 1 tbsp. olive oil
- ½ tbsp. apple cider
- ½ tsp. brown Swerve

Directions:

1. Put all the salad ingredients into a suitable salad bowl.
2. Toss them well and refrigerate for 1 h.
3. Serve.

Nutrition - Per Serving: Calories: 173; Fat 7.1g; Sodium 80mg; Protein 1.6g; Calcium 50mg; Phosphorous 96mg; Potassium 501mg

271.   BUTTERSCOTCH APPLE SALAD

Preparation Time: 5 min.   **Cooking Time:** 0 min.   **Servings**: 6

Ingredients:

- 3 cups jazz apples, chopped
- 8 oz. canned crushed pineapple
- 8 oz. whipped topping
- 1/2 cup butterscotch topping
- 1/3 cup almonds
- 1/4 cup butterscotch chips

Directions:

1. Put all the salad ingredients into a suitable salad bowl.
2. Toss them well and refrigerate for 1 h.
3. Serve.

Nutrition: Calories: 293; Fat 12.7g; Sodium 52mg; Protein 4.2g; Calcium 65mg; Phosphorous 202mg; Potassium 296mg

272.   CRANBERRY CABBAGE SLAW

Preparation Time: 5 min.   **Cooking Time:** 0 min.   **Servings**: 4

Ingredients:

- 1/2 medium cabbage head, shredded
- 1 medium red apple, shredded
- 2 tbsp. onion, sliced
- 1/2 cup dried cranberries
- 1/4 cup almonds, toasted sliced
- 1/2 cup olive oil
- ¼ tsp. stevia
- 1/4 cup cider vinegar
- 1/2 tbsp. celery seed
- 1/2 tsp. dry mustard
- ½ cup cream

Directions:

1. Take a suitable salad bowl.
2. Start tossing in all the ingredients.
3. Mix well and serve.

Nutrition: Calories: 308; Fat 24.5g; Sodium 23mg; Protein 2.6g; Calcium 69mg; Phosphorous 257mg; Potassium 219mg

273.   CHESTNUT NOODLE SALAD

Preparation Time: 5 min.   **Cooking Time:** 0 min.   **Servings**: 6

Ingredients:

- 8 cups cabbage, shredded
- 1/2 cup canned chestnuts, sliced
- 6 green onions, chopped
- 1/4 cup olive oil
- 1/4 cup apple cider vinegar
- 3/4 tsp. stevia
- 1/8 tsp. black pepper
- 1 cup chow Mein noodles, cooked

Directions:

1. Take a suitable salad bowl.
2. Start tossing in all the ingredients.
3. Mix well and serve.

Nutrition - Per Serving: Calories: 191; Fat 13g; Cholesterol 1mg; Sodium 78mg; Protein 4.2g; Calcium 142mg; Phosphorous 188mg; Potassium 302mg

CHAPTER 14. DRINKS AND JUICES

274. ALMONDS & BLUEBERRIES SMOOTHIE

Preparation Time: 5 min.   **Cooking Time:** 3 min.   **Servings**: 2

Ingredients:

- 1/4 cup ground almonds, unsalted
- 1 cup fresh blueberries
- Fresh juice of a 1 lemon
- 1 cup fresh kale leaf
- 1/2 cup coconut water
- 1 cup water
- 2 tbsp. plain yogurt (optional)

Directions:

1. Dump all ingredients in your high-speed blender, and blend until your smoothie is smooth.
2. Pour the mixture in a chilled glass.
3. Serve and enjoy!

Nutrition: Calories: 110; Carbs: 8g; Proteins: 2g; Fat: 7g; Fiber: 2g; Sodium: 1mg; Potassium: 174mg

275. ALMONDS AND ZUCCHINI SMOOTHIE

Preparation Time: 5 min.   **Cooking Time:** 3 min.   **Servings**: 2

Ingredients:

- 1 cup zucchini, cooked and mashed - unsalted
- 1 1/2 cups almond milk
- 1 tbsp. almond butter (plain, unsalted)
- 1 tsp. pure almond extract
- 2 tbsp. ground almonds or macadamia almonds
- 1/2 cup water
- 1 cup ice cubes crushed (optional, for serving)

Directions:

1. Dump all ingredients from the list above in your fast-speed blender; blend for 45 - 60 seconds, or taste.
2. Serve with crushed ice.

Nutrition: Calories: 322; Carbs: 6g; Proteins: 6g; Fat: 30g; Fiber: 3.5g; Sodium: 35mg; Potassium: 726mg

276. AVOCADO WITH WALNUT BUTTER SMOOTHIE

Preparation Time: 5 min.   **Cooking Time:** 3 min.   **Servings**: 2

Ingredients:

- 1 avocado (diced)
- 1 cup baby spinach
- 1 cup coconut milk (canned)
- 1 tbsp. walnut butter, unsalted
- 2 tbsp. natural sweetener such as stevia, erythritol, truvia...etc

Directions:

1. Place all ingredients into food processor or a blender; blend until smooth or to taste.
2. Add more or less walnut butter.
3. Drink and enjoy!

Nutrition - Per Serving: Calories: 364; Carbs: 7g; Proteins: 8g; Fat: 35g; Fiber: 5.5g; Sodium: 36mg; Potassium: 887mg

277. BABY SPINACH AND DILL SMOOTHIE

Preparation Time: 5 min.   **Cooking Time:** 3 min.   **Servings**: 2

Ingredients:

- 1 cup of fresh baby spinach leaves
- 2 tbsp. of fresh dill, chopped
- 1 1/2 cup of water
- 1/2 avocado, chopped into cubes
- 1 tbsp. chia seeds (optional)
- 2 tbsp. of natural sweetener stevia or erythritol (optional)

Directions:

1. Place all ingredients into fast-speed blender. Beat until smooth and all ingredients united well.
2. Serve and enjoy!

Nutrition - Per Serving: Calories: 136; Carbs: 8g; Proteins: 7g; Fat: 10g; Fiber: 9g; Sodium: 29mg; Potassium: 489mg

278.   BLUEBERRIES AND COCONUT SMOOTHIE

Preparation Time: 5 min.   **Cooking Time:** 3 min.   **Servings**: 5

Ingredients:

- 1 cup of frozen blueberries, unsweetened
- 1 cup stevia or erythritol sweetener
- 2 cups coconut milk (canned)
- 1 cup of fresh spinach leaves
- 2 tbsp. shredded coconut (unsweetened)
- 3/4 cup water

Directions:

1. Place all ingredients from the list in food-processor or in your strong blender.
2. Blend for 45 - 60 seconds or to taste.
3. Ready for drink! Serve!

Nutrition: Calories: 190; Carbs: 8g; Proteins: 3g; Fat: 18g; Fiber: 2g; Sodium: 20mg; Potassium: 315mg

279.   COLLARD GREENS AND CUCUMBER SMOOTHIE

Preparation Time: 15 min.   **Cooking Time:** 5 min.   **Servings**: 2

Ingredients:

- 1 cup collard greens
- A few fresh pepper mint leaves
- 1 big cucumber
- 1 lime, freshly juiced
- 1/2 cups avocado sliced
- 1 1/2 cup water
- 1 cup crushed ice
- 1/4 cup of natural sweetener erythritol or stevia (optional)

Directions:

1. Rinse and clean your collard greens from any dirt.
2. Blend all ingredients in a blender until your smoothie is combined well.
3. Pour in a glass and drink. Enjoy!

Nutrition: Calories: 123; Carbs: 8g; Proteins: 4g; Fat: 11g; Fiber: 6g; Sodium: 10mg; Potassium: 432mg

280.   CREAMY DANDELION GREENS AND CELERY SMOOTHIE

Preparation Time: 10 min.   **Cooking Time:** 3 min.   **Servings**: 2

Ingredients:

- 1 handful of raw dandelion greens
- 2 celery sticks
- 2 tbsp. chia seeds
- 1 small piece of ginger, minced
- 1/2 cup almond milk
- 1/2 cup of water
- 1/2 cup plain yogurt

Directions:

1. Rinse and clean dandelion leaves from any dirt; add in a high-speed blender. Clean the ginger; keep only inner part and cut in small slices; add in a blender.
2. Blend all remaining ingredients until smooth.
3. Serve and enjoy!

Nutrition: Calories: 58; Carbs: 5g; Proteins: 3g; Fat: 6g; Fiber: 3g; Sodium: 116mg; Potassium: 630mg

281.   DARK TURNIP GREENS SMOOTHIE

Preparation Time: 10 min.   **Cooking Time:** 3 min.   **Servings**: 2

Ingredients:

- 1 cup of raw turnip greens
- 1 1/2 cup of almond milk
- 1 tbsp. of almond butter
- 1/2 cup of water
- 1/2 tsp. of cocoa powder, unsweetened
- 1 tbsp. of dark chocolate chips
- 1/4 tsp. of cinnamon
- A pinch of salt
- 1/2 cup of crushed ice

Directions:

1. Rinse and clean turnip greens from any dirt.
2. Place the turnip greens in your blender along with all other ingredients.
3. Blend it for 45 - 60 seconds or until done; smooth and creamy.
4. Serve with or without crushed ice.

Nutrition: Calories: 131; Carbs: 6g; Proteins: 4g; Fat: 10g; Fiber: 2.5g; Sodium: 40mg; Potassium: 627mg

282.   BUTTER PECAN AND COCONUT SMOOTHIE

Preparation Time: 5 min.   **Cooking Time:** 2 min.   **Servings**: 2

Ingredients:

- 1 cup coconut milk, canned
- 1 scoop butter pecan powdered creamer
- 2 cups fresh spinach leaves, chopped
- 1/2 banana frozen or fresh
- 2 tbsp. stevia granulated sweetener to taste
- 1/2 cup water
- 1 cup ice cubes crushed

Directions:

1. Place ingredients from the list above in your high-speed blender.
2. Blend for 35 - 50 seconds or until all ingredients combined well.
3. Add less or more crushed ice.
4. Drink and enjoy!

Nutrition - Per Serving: Calories: 268; Carbs: 7g; Proteins: 6g; Fat: 26g; Fiber: 1.5g; Sodium: 50mg; Potassium: 561mg

283.   FRESH CUCUMBER, KALE AND RASPBERRY SMOOTHIE

Preparation Time: 10 min.   **Cooking Time:** 3 min.   **Servings**: 3

Ingredients:

- 1 1/2 cups of cucumber, peeled
- 1/2 cup raw kale leaves
- 1 1/2 cups fresh raspberries
- 1 cup of almond milk
- 1 cup of water
- Ice cubes crushed (optional)
- 2 tbsp. natural sweetener (stevia, erythritol...etc.)

Directions:

1   Place all Ingredients listed in a High-Speed Blender; Blend For 35 - 40 Seconds.

2   Serve into Chilled Glasses.

3   Add More Natural Sweeter if you like. Enjoy!

Nutrition - Per Serv: Calories: 70; Carbs: 8g; Proteins: 3g; Fat: 6g; Fiber: 5g; Sodium: 19mg; Potassium: 435mg

284.   FRESH LETTUCE AND CUCUMBER-LEMON SMOOTHIE

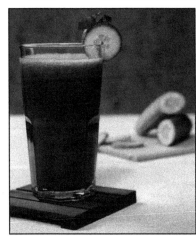

Preparation Time: 10 min.

Cooking Time: 3 min.

Servings: 2

Nutrition - Per Serving:

Calories: 51

Carbs: 4g

Proteins: 2g

Fat: 4g

Fiber: 3.5g

Sodium: 18mg

Potassium: 555mg

Ingredients:

- 2 cups fresh lettuce leaves, chopped (any kind)
- 1 cup of cucumber
- 1 lemon washed and sliced.
- 1/2 avocado
- 2 tbsp. chia seeds
- 1 1/2 cup water or coconut water
- 1/4 cup stevia granulate sweetener (or to taste)

Directions:

1. Add all ingredients from the list above in the high-speed blender, blend until completely smooth.
2. Pour your smoothie into chilled glasses and enjoy!

CHAPTER 15. SMOOTHIES

285. FRUITY SMOOTHIE

Preparation Time: 10min. **Cooking Time:** 0 min. **Servings:** 2

Ingredients:

- 8 oz canned fruits, with juice
- 2 scoops vanilla-flavored whey protein powder
- 1 cup cold water
- 1 cup crushed ice

Directions:

1. First, start by putting all the ingredients in a blender jug.
2. Give it a pulse for 30 seconds until blended well. Serve chilled and fresh.

Nutrition - Per Serving: Calories: 186; Protein 23 g; Fat 2g; Cholesterol 41 mg; Potassium 282 mg; Calcium 160 mg; Fiber 1.1 g; Sodium: 6mg

286. MIXED BERRY PROTEIN SMOOTHIE

Preparation Time: 10min. **Cooking Time:** 0 min. **Servings:** 2

Ingredients:

- 4 oz cold water
- 1 cup frozen mixed berries
- 2 ice cubes
- 1 tsp. blueberry essence
- 1/2 cup whipped cream topping
- 2 scoops whey protein powder

Directions:

1. First, start by putting all the ingredients in a blender jug.
2. Give it a pulse for 30 seconds until blended well. Serve chilled and fresh.

Nutrition - Per Serving: Calories: 104; Protein 6 g; Fat 4 g; Cholesterol 11 mg; Potassium 141 mg; Calcium 69 mg; Fiber 2.4 g; Sodium: 57mg

287. PEACH HIGH-PROTEIN SMOOTHIE

Preparation Time: 10min. **Cooking Time:** 0 min. **Servings:** 1

Ingredients:

- 1/2 cup ice
- 2 tbsp. powdered egg whites
- 3/4 cup fresh peaches
- 1 tbsp. sugar

Directions:

1. First, start by putting all the ingredients in a blender jug.
2. Give it a pulse for 30 seconds until blended well. Serve chilled and fresh.

Nutrition - Per Serving: Calories: 132; Protein 10 g; Fat 0 g; Cholesterol 0 mg; Potassium 353 mg; Calcium 9 mg; Fiber 1.9 g; Sodium: 347mg

288. STRAWBERRY FRUIT SMOOTHIE

Preparation Time: 10min. **Cooking Time:** 0 min. **Servings:** 1

Ingredients:

- 3/4 cup fresh strawberries
- 1/2 cup liquid pasteurized egg whites
- 1/2 cup ice
- 1 tbsp. sugar

Directions:

1. First, start by putting all the ingredients in a blender jug.
2. Give it a pulse for 30 seconds until blended well. Serve chilled and fresh.

Nutrition - Per Serving: Calories: 156; Protein 14 g; Fat 0 g; Cholesterol 0 mg; Potassium 400 mg; Phosphorus 49 mg; Calcium 29 mg; Fiber 2.5 g; Sodium: 42mg

---

289. WATERMELON BLISS

Preparation Time: 10min. **Cooking Time:** 0 min. **Servings**: 2

Ingredients:

- 2 cups watermelon
- 1 medium-sized cucumber, peeled and sliced
- 2 mint sprigs, leaves only
- 1 celery stalk
- Squeeze of lime juice

Directions:

1. First, start by putting all the ingredients in a blender jug.
2. Give it a pulse for 30 seconds until blended well. Serve chilled and fresh.

Nutrition - Per Serving: Calories: 156; Protein 14 g; Fat 0 g; Cholesterol 0 mg; Potassium 400 mg; Calcium 29 mg; Fiber 2.5g; Sodium: 55mg

---

290. CRANBERRY SMOOTHIE

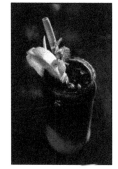

Preparation Time: 10min.

Cooking Time: 0 min.

Servings: 1

Nutrition - Per Serving:

Calories: 126	Potassium 220 mg
Protein 12 g	Calcium 19 mg
Fat 0.03 g	Fiber 1.4g
Cholesterol 0 mg	Sodium: 88mg

Ingredients:

- 1 cup frozen cranberries
- 1 medium cucumber, peeled and sliced
- 1 stalk of celery
- Handful of parsley
- Squeeze of lime juice

Directions:

1. First, start by putting all the ingredients in a blender jug. Give it a pulse for 30 seconds until blended well.
2. Serve chilled and fresh.

---

291. BERRY CUCUMBER SMOOTHIE

Preparation Time: 10min. **Cooking Time:** 0 min. **Servings**: 1

Ingredients:

- 1 medium cucumber, peeled and sliced
- ½ cup fresh blueberries
- ½ cup fresh or frozen strawberries
- ½ cup unsweetened rice milk
- Stevia, to taste

Directions:

1. First, start by putting all the ingredients in a blender jug.
2. Give it a pulse for 30 seconds until blended well.
3. Serve chilled and fresh.

Nutrition: Calories: 141; Protein 1 g; Carbs 15g; Fat 0g; Sodium 113mg; Potassium 230mg; Phosphorus 129 mg

292. RASPBERRY PEACH SMOOTHIE

Preparation Time: 10min.　　**Cooking Time:** 0 min.　　**Servings:** 2

Ingredients:

- 1 cup frozen raspberries
- 1 medium peach, pit removed, sliced
- ½ cup silken tofu
- 1 tbsp. honey
- 1 cup unsweetened vanilla almond milk

Directions:

1. First, start by putting all the ingredients in a blender jug.
2. Give it a pulse for 30 seconds until blended well.
3. Serve chilled and fresh.

Nutrition - Per Serving: Calories: 132; Protein 9 g; Fat: 0 g; Carbs 14 g; Sodium 112 mg; Potassium 310 mg; Phosphorus 39 mg; Calcium 32 mg

293. POWER-BOOSTING SMOOTHIE

Preparation Time: 5 min.　　**Cooking Time:** 0 min.　　**Servings:** 2

Ingredients:

- ½ cup water
- ½ cup non-dairy whipped topping
- 2 scoops whey protein powder
- 1½ cups frozen blueberries

Directions:

1. In a high-speed blender, add all ingredients and pulse till smooth.
2. Transfer into 2 serving glass and serve immediately.

Nutrition - Per Serving: Calories: 242; Fat 7g; Carbs 23.8g; Protein: 23.2g; Potassium: 263mg; Sodium: 63mg; Phosphorous: 30 mg

294. DISTINCTIVE PINEAPPLE SMOOTHIE

Preparation Time: 5 min.　　**Cooking Time:** 0 min.　　**Servings:** 2

Ingredients:

- ¼ cup crushed ice cubes
- 2 scoops vanilla whey protein powder
- 1 cup water
- 1½ cups pineapple

Directions:

1. In a high-speed blender, add all ingredients and pulse till smooth.
2. Transfer into 2 serving glass and serve immediately.

Nutrition - Per Serving: Calories: 117; Fat: 2.1g; Carbs: 18.2g; Protein: 22.7g; Potassium: 296mg; Sodium:81mg; Phosphorous: 28 mg

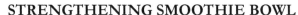

295.   STRENGTHENING SMOOTHIE BOWL

Preparation Time: 5 min.   **Cooking Time:** 4 min.   **Servings**: 2

Ingredients:

- ¼ cup fresh blueberries
- ¼ cup fat-free plain Greek yogurt
- 1/3 cup unsweetened almond milk
- 2 tbsp. of whey protein powder
- 2 cups frozen blueberries

Directions:

1. In a blender, add blueberries and pulse for about 1 min.
2. Add almond milk, yogurt and protein powder and pulse till desired consistency.
3. Transfer the mixture into 2 bowls evenly.
4. Serve with the topping of fresh blueberries.

Nutrition - Per Serving: Calories: 176; Fat 2.1g; Carbs 27g; Protein 15.1g; Potassium: 242mg; Sodium: 72mg; Phosphorous 555.3 mg

296.   PINEAPPLE JUICE

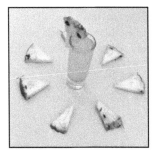

Preparation Time: 5 min.

Cooking Time: 0 min.

Servings: 2

Nutrition - Per Serving:

Calories: 135

Protein: 0 g; Carbs: 0 g; Fat: 0 g

Sodium: 0 mg; Potassium:180 mg; Phosphorus 8 mg

Ingredients:

- ½ cup canned pineapple
- 1 cup water

Directions:

1. Blend all ingredients and serve over ice.

297.   GRAPEFRUIT SORBET

Preparation Time: 10 min.   **Cooking Time:** 5 min.   **Servings**: 6

Ingredients:

- ½ cup sugar
- ¼ cup water
- 1 fresh thyme sprig
- For the sorbet
- Juice of 6 pink grapefruit
- ¼ cup thyme simple syrup
- To make the thyme simple syrup
- In a small saucepan, combine the sugar, water, and thyme. Bring to a boil, turn off the heat, and refrigerate, thyme sprig included, until cold. Strain the thyme sprig from the syrup.
- To make the sorbet

Directions:

1. In a blender, combine the grapefruit juice and ¼ cup of simple syrup, and process.
2. Transfer to an airtight container and freeze for 3 to 4 hs, until firm. Serve.
3. Substitution tip: Try this with other citrus fruits, such as oranges, lemons, or limes, for an equally delicious treat.

Nutrition - Per Serving: Calories: 117; Fat 2.1g; Carbs 18.2g; Protein 22.7g; Potassium: 296mg; Sodium: 81mg; Phosphorous 28 mg

---

298.   APPLE AND BLUEBERRY CRISP

Preparation Time: 1 h 10 min   **Cooking Time:** 1 h   **Servings:** 8

Ingredients:

- Crisp
- 1/4 cup of brown sugar
- 1 1/4 cups quick cooking rolled oats

FILLING:

- 2 tbsp. cornstarch
- 1/2 cup of brown sugar
- 2 cups chopped or grated apples

- 6 tbsp. non-hydrogenated melted margarine
- 1/4 cup all-purpose flour (unbleached)

- cups frozen or fresh blueberries (not thawed)
- 1 tbsp. fresh lemon juice
- 1 tbsp. melted margarine

Directions:

1. Preheat the oven to 350°F with the rack in the middle position.
2. Pour all the dry ingredients into a bowl, then the butter and stir until it is moistened. Set the mixture aside. In an 8-inch (20-cm) square baking dish, mix the cornstarch and brown sugar. Add lemon juice and the rest of the fruits. Toss to blend the mixture. Add the crisp mixture, then bake until the crisp turns golden brown (or for 55 min. to 1 h). You can either serve cold or warm.

Nutrition - Per Serving: Calories: 127; Fat 2.1g; Carbs 18.2g; Protein 22.7g; Potassium 256mg; Sodium 61mg; Phosphorous 28 mg

---

299.   COCONUT BREAKFAST SMOOTHIE

Preparation Time: 5 min.   **Cooking Time:** 5 min.   **Servings:** 1

Ingredients:

- 1/4 cup whey protein powder
- 1/2 cup coconut milk
- 5 drops liquid stevia
- tbsp. coconut oil
- tsp. vanilla
- tbsp. coconut butter
- 1/4 cup water
- 1/2 cup ice

Directions:

1. Add all ingredients into the blender and blend until smooth.
2. Serve and enjoy.

Nutrition: Calories 560 Fat 45g Carbs 12g Sugar 4g Protein 25g Cholesterol 60 mg

CHAPTER 16. DESSERT RECIPES

300.   CHOCOLATE TRIFLE

Preparation Time: 20 min.   **Cooking Time:** 15 min.   **Servings**: 4

Ingredients:

- 1 small plain sponge Swiss roll
- oz. custard powder
- oz. hot water
- 16 oz. canned mandarins
- tbsp. sherry
- oz. double cream
- 4 chocolate squares, grated

Directions:

1. Whisk the custard powder with water in a bowl until dissolved. In a bowl, mix the custard well until it becomes creamy and let it sit for 15 min. Spread the Swiss roll and cut it in 4 squares.
2. Place the Swiss roll in the 4 serving cups.
3. Top the Swiss roll with mandarin, custard, cream, and chocolate.
4. Serve.

Nutrition - Per Serving: Calories: 315; Fat 13.5g; Cholesterol 43mg; Sodium 185mg; Protein 2.9g; Calcium 61mg; Phosphorous 184mg; Potassium 129mg

301.   PINEAPPLE MERINGUES

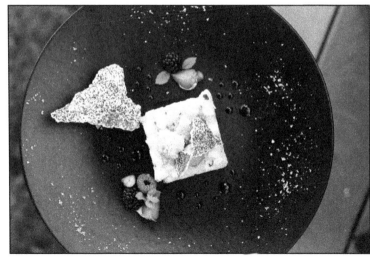

Preparation Time: 10 min.

Cooking Time: 0 min.

Servings: 4

Nutrition - Per Serving:

Calories: 312

Cholesterol 0mg

Sodium 41mg

Protein 2.3g

Calcium 3mg

Phosphorous 104mg

Potassium 110mg

Ingredients:

- meringue nests
- oz. crème fraiche
- 2 oz. stem ginger, chopped
- oz. can pineapple chunks

Directions:

1. Place the meringue nests on the serving plates.
2. Whisk the ginger with crème Fraiche and pineapple chunks.
3. Divide this the pineapple mixture over the meringue nests.
4. Serve.

302. BAKED CUSTARD

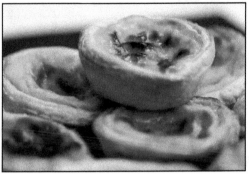

Preparation Time: 15 min.

Cooking Time: 30 min.

Servings: 1

Nutrition - Per Serving:

Calories: 127

Fat 7g; Cholesterol 174mg

Sodium 119mg; Calcium 169mg

Phosphorous 309mg; Potassium 171mg

Ingredients:

- 1/2 cup milk
- 1 egg, beaten
- 1/8 tsp. nutmeg
- 1/8 tsp. vanilla
- Sweetener, to taste
- 1/2 cup water

Directions:

1. Lightly warm up the milk in a pan, then whisk in the egg, nutmeg, vanilla and sweetener.
2. Pour this custard mixture into a ramekin.
3. Place the ramekin in a baking pan and pour ½ cup water into the pan.
4. Bake the custard for 30 min. at 325 F. Serve fresh.

303. STRAWBERRY PIE

Preparation Time: 15 min.   **Cooking Time:** 25 min.   **Servings**: 6

Ingredients:

- 1 unbaked (9 inches) pie shell
- cups strawberries, fresh
- 1 cup of brown Swerve
- tbsp. arrowroot powder
- 2 tbsp. lemon juice
- tbsp. whipped cream topping

Directions:

1. Spread the pie shell in the pie pan and bake it until golden brown.
2. Now mash 2 cups of strawberries with the lemon juice, arrowroot powder, and Swerve in a bowl. Add the mixture to a saucepan and cook on moderate heat until it thickens.
3. Allow the mixture to cool then spread it in the pie shell.
4. Slice the remaining strawberries and spread them over the pie filling.
5. Refrigerate for 1 h then garnish with whipped cream. Serve fresh and enjoy.

Nutrition - Per Serving: Calories: 236; Fat 11.1g; Cholesterol 3mg; Sodium 183mg; Protein 2.2g; Calcium 23mg; Phosphorous 47.2mg; Potassium 178mg

304. APPLE CRISP

Preparation Time: 20 min.   **Cooking Time:** 45 min.   **Servings**: 6

Ingredients:

- cups apples, peeled and chopped
- ½ tsp. stevia
- tbsp. brandy
- 2 tsp. lemon juice
- 1/2 tsp. cinnamon
- 1/8 tsp. nutmeg
- 3/4 cup dry oats
- 1/4 cup brown Swerve
- 2 tbsp. flour
- 2 tbsp. butter

Directions:

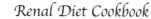
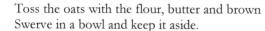
1. Toss the oats with the flour, butter and brown Swerve in a bowl and keep it aside.
2. Whisk the remaining crisp ingredients in an 8-inch baking pan.
3. Spread the oats mixture over the crispy filling.
4. Bake it for 45 min. at 350 F in a preheated oven.
5. Slice and serve.

Nutrition - Per Serving: Calories: 214; Fat 4.8g; Cholesterol 0mg; Sodium 48mg; Protein 2.1g; Calcium 15mg; Phosphorous 348mg; Potassium 212mg

305. ALMOND COOKIES

Preparation Time: 10 min.   **Cooking Time:** 12 min.   **Servings**: 24

Ingredients:

- 1 cup butter, softened
- 1 cup granulate Swerve
- 1 egg
- cups flour
- 1 tsp. baking soda
- 1 tsp. almond extract

Directions:

1. Beat the butter with the Swerve in a mixer then gradually stir in the remaining ingredients.
2. Mix well until it forms a cookie dough then divide the dough into small balls.
3. Spread each ball into ¾ inch rounds and place them in a cookie sheet.
4. Poke 2-3 holes in each cookie then bake for 12 min. at 400 F. Serve.

Nutrition - Per Serving: Calories: 159; Fat 7.9g; Cholesterol 7mg; Sodium 144mg; Protein 1.9g; Calcium 6mg; Phosphorous 274mg; Potassium 23mg

306. LIME PIE

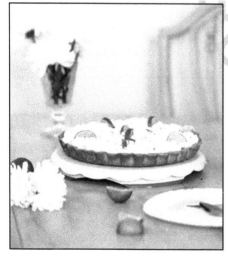

Preparation Time: 10 min.

Cooking Time: 5 min.

Servings: 8

Nutrition - Per Serving:

Calories: 391

Total Fat 22.4g

Cholesterol 57mg

Sodium 52mg

Protein 5.3g

Calcium 163mg

Phosphorous 199mg

Potassium 221mg

Ingredients:

- tbsp. butter, unsalted
- 1 1/4 cups breadcrumbs
- 1/4 cup granulated Swerve
- 1/3 cup lime juice
- 14 oz. condensed milk
- 1 cup heavy whipping cream
- 1 (9 inches) pie shell

Directions:

1. Switch on your gas oven and preheat it to 350 F. Whisk the cracker crumbs with the Swerve and melted butter in a suitable bowl.
2. Spread this cracker crumbs crust in a 9 inches pie shell and bake it for 5 min.
3. Meanwhile, mix the condensed milk with the lime juice in a bowl.
4. Whisk the heavy cream in a mixer until foamy, then add in the condensed milk mixture.
5. Mix well, then spread this filling in the baked crust.
6. Refrigerate the pie for 4 hs.
7. Slice and serve.

307. BUTTERY LEMON SQUARES

Preparation Time: 10 min.   **Cooking Time:** 35 min.   **Servings:** 12

Ingredients:

- 1 cup refined Swerve
- 1 cup flour
- 1/2 cup butter, unsalted
- 1 cup granulated Swerve
- 1/2 tsp. baking powder
- 2 eggs, beaten
- tbsp. lemon juice
- 1 tbsp. butter, unsalted, softened
- 1 tbsp. lemon zest

Directions:

1. Start mixing ¼ cup refined Swerve, ½ cup butter, and flour in a bowl.
2. Spread this crust mixture in an 8-inch square pan and press it.
3. Bake this flour crust for 15 min. at 350 F.
4. Meanwhile, prepare the filling by beating 2 tbsp. lemon juice, granulated Swerve, eggs, lemon rind, and baking powder in a mixer.
5. Spread this filling in the baked crust and bake again for about 20 min.
6. Meanwhile, prepare the squares' icing by beating 2 tbsp. lemon juice, 1 tbsp. butter, and ¾ cup refine Swerve.
7. Once the lemon pie is baked well, allow it to cool.
8. Sprinkle the icing mixture on top of the lemon pie then cut it into 36 squares. Serve.

Nutrition - Per Serving: Calories: 229; Fat 9.5g; Cholesterol 50mg; Sodium 66mg; Protein 2.1g; Calcium 18mg; Phosphorous 257mg; Potassium 51mg

308. BLACKBERRY CREAM CHEESE PIE

Preparation Time: 15 min.   **Cooking Time:** 45 min.   **Servings:** 8

Ingredients:

- 1/3 cup butter, unsalted
- cups blackberries
- 1 tsp. stevia
- 1 cup flour
- 1/2 tsp. baking powder
- 3/4 cup cream cheese

Directions:

1. Switch your gas oven to 375 F to preheat. Layer a 2-quart baking dish with melted butter.
2. Mix the blackberries with stevia in a small bowl. Beat the remaining ingredients in a mixer until they form a smooth batter.
3. Evenly spread this pie batter in the prepared baking dish and top it with blackberries.
4. Bake the blackberry pie for about 45 min. in the preheated oven.
5. Slice and serve once chilled.

Nutrition - Per Serving: Calories: 239; Fat 8.4g; Cholesterol 20mg; Sodium 63mg; Protein 2.8g; Calcium 67mg; Phosphorous 105mg; Potassium 170mg

309. MAPLE CRISP BARS

Preparation Time: 10 min.   **Cooking Time:** 5 min.   **Servings:** 20

Ingredients:

- 1/3 cup butter
- 1 cup brown Swerve
- 1 tsp. maple extract
- 1/2 cup maple syrup
- cups puffed rice cereal

Directions:

1   Mix the butter with Swerve, maple extract, and syrup in a saucepan over moderate heat.
2   Cook by slowly stirring this mixture for 5 min. then toss in the rice cereal.
3   Mix well, then press this cereal mixture in a 13x9 inches baking dish.
4   Refrigerate the mixture for 2 hs then cut into 20 bars.
5   Serve.

Nutrition - Per Serving: Calories: 107; Fat 3.1g; Cholesterol 0mg; Sodium 36mg; Protein 0.4g; Calcium 7mg; Phosphorous 233mg; Potassium 24mg

310.   PINEAPPLE GELATIN PIE

Preparation Time: 10 min.   **Cooking Time:** 5 min.   **Servings**: 8

Ingredients:

- 2/3 cup graham cracker crumbs
- 1/2 tbsp. butter, melted
- 1 (20-oz) can crushed pineapple, juice packed
- 1 small gelatin pack
- 1 tbsp. lemon juice
- 2 egg whites, pasteurized
- 1/4 tsp. cream of tartar

Directions:

1   Whisk the crumbs with the butter in a bowl then spread them onto an 8-inch pie plate.
2   Bake the crust for 5 min. at 425 F.
3   Meanwhile, mix the pineapple juice with the gelatin in a saucepan.
4   Place it over low heat then add the pineapple and lemon juice. Mix well.
5   Beat the cream of tartar and egg whites in a mixer until creamy. Add the cooked pineapple mixture then mix well.
6   Spread this filling in the baked crust.
7   Refrigerate the pie for 4 hs then slice.
8   Serve.

Nutrition - Per Serving: Calories: 106; Fat 4.2g; Cholesterol 0mg; Sodium 117mg; Protein 2.2g; Calcium 3mg; Phosphorous 231mg; Potassium 33mg

311.   CHOCOLATE GELATIN MOUSSE

Preparation Time: 10 min.   **Cooking Time:** 5 min.   **Servings**: 4

Ingredients:

- 1 tsp. stevia
- 1/2 tsp. gelatin
- 1/4 cup milk
- 1/2 cup chocolate chips
- 1 tsp. vanilla
- 1/2 cup heavy cream, whipped

Directions:

1   Whisk the stevia with the gelatin and milk in a saucepan and cook up to a boil.
2   Stir in the chocolate and vanilla then mix well until it has completely melted.
3   Beat the cream in a mixer until fluffy then fold in the chocolate mixture.
4   Mix it gently with a spatula then transfer to the serving bowl.
5   Refrigerate the dessert for 4 hs.
6   Serve.

Nutrition - Per Serving: Calories: 200; Fat 12.1g; Cholesterol 27mg; Sodium 31mg; Protein 3.2g; Calcium 68mg; Phosphorous 120mg; Potassium 100mg

312. CHEESECAKE BITES

Preparation Time: 10 min.   **Cooking Time:** 5 min.   **Servings**: 16

Ingredients:

- 8 oz cream cheese
- 1/2 tsp. vanilla
- 1/4 cup swerve

Directions:

1. Add all ingredients into the mixing bowl and blend until well combined.
2. Place bowl into the fridge for 1 h.
3. Remove bowl from the fridge. Make small balls from cheese mixture and place them on a baking dish.
4. Serve and enjoy.

Nutrition - Per Serving: Calories: 50 Fat 4.9 g Carbs 0.4 g Sugar 0.1 g Protein 1.1 g Cholesterol 16 mg Phosphorus: 110mg Potassium: 117mg Sodium: 75mg

313. PUMPKIN BITES

Preparation Time: 10 min.   **Cooking Time:** 5 min.   **Servings**: 12

Ingredients:

- 8 oz cream cheese
- 1 tsp. vanilla
- 1 tsp. pumpkin pie spice
- 1/4 cup coconut flour
- 1/4 cup erythritol
- 1/2 cup pumpkin puree
- 4 oz butter

Directions:

1. Add all ingredients into the mixing bowl and beat using hand mixer until well combined.
2. Scoop mixture into the silicone ice cube tray and place it in the refrigerator until set. Serve and enjoy.

Nutrition - Per Serving: Calories: 149 Fat 14.6 g Carbs 8.1 g Sugar 5.4 g Protein 2 g Cholesterol 41 mg Phosphorus: 66mg Potassium: 77mg Sodium: 55mg

314. PROTEIN BALLS

Preparation Time: 5 min.   **Cooking Time:** 5 min.   **Servings**: 12

Ingredients:

- 3/4 cup peanut butter
- 1 tsp. cinnamon
- 3 tbsp. erythritol
- 1 1/2 cup almond flour

Directions:

1. Add all ingredients into the mixing bowl and blend until well combined.
2. Place bowl into the fridge for 30 min.
3. Remove bowl from the fridge. Make small balls from mixture and place on a baking dish. Serve and enjoy.

Nutrition - Per Serving: Calories: 179 Fat 14.8 g Carbs 10.1 g Sugar 5.3 g Protein 7 g Cholesterol 0 mg Phosphorus: 70mg Potassium: 87mg Sodium:95mg

315. CHOCOLATE MOUSSE

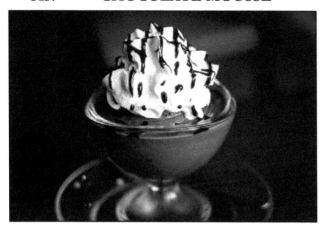

Preparation Time: 5 min.
Cooking Time: 5 min.
Servings: 4
Nutrition - Per Serving:
Calories: 255
Fat 24 g
Carbs 6 g
Sugar 0.5 g
Protein 5.1 g
Cholesterol 80 mg
Phosphorus: 110mg
Potassium: 117mg
Sodium: 75mg

Ingredients:

- 1/2 cup unsweetened cocoa powder
- 1/2 tsp. vanilla
- 1 1/4 cup heavy cream
- 4 oz cream cheese
- 8 drops liquid stevia

Directions:

1. Add all ingredients into the blender and blend until smooth and creamy.
2. Pour mixture into the serving bowls and place in the refrigerator for 1-2 hs.
3. Serve and enjoy.

316. ALMOND BITES

Preparation Time: 10 min.   **Cooking Time:** 10 min.   **Servings:** 12

Ingredients:

- 1/2 cup almond meal
- 2 tbsp. coconut butter
- dates, pitted and chopped
- 1/4 cup unsweetened chocolate chips
- 1/2 tsp. vanilla

Directions:

1. Add dates in the food processor and process for 30 seconds.
2. Add remaining ingredients except chocolate chips and process until combined.
3. Add chocolate chips and process for 15 seconds.
4. Make small balls from mixture and place on a baking tray. Place in refrigerator for 1-2 hs. Serve and enjoy

Nutrition - Per Serving: Calories: 53 Fat 3.8 g Carbs 4.2 g Sugar 2.2 g Protein 1.1 g Cholesterol 1 mg Phosphorus: 110mg Potassium: 117mg Sodium: 75mg

317. HEALTHY PROTEIN BARS

Preparation Time: 10 min.   **Cooking Time:** 10 min.   **Servings:** 8

Ingredients:

- 2 scoops vanilla protein powder
- 1/4 cup coconut oil, melted
- 1 cup almond butter
- 1 tsp. cinnamon
- 18 drops liquid stevia
- Pinch of salt

Directions:

1. Add all ingredients into the mixing bowl and mix until well combined.
2. Pour mixture into the baking dish and spread evenly.

3. Place in refrigerator for 2-3 hs.
4. Slice and serve.

Nutrition - Per Serving: Calories: 99 Fat 8 g Carbs 0.7 g Sugar 0.2 g Protein 7.2 g Cholesterol 0 mg Phosphorus: 85mg Potassium: 97mg Sodium: 105mg

318.   ORANGE AND CINNAMON BISCOTTI

Preparation Time: 1 h 20 min.   **Cooking Time:** 1h   **Servings**: 18 cookies

Ingredients
- ½ cup butter, unsalted, room temperature
- 1 cup sugar
- 2 tsp. orange peel, grated
- 2 large eggs
- 2 cups flour, all-purpose
- 1 tsp. Vanilla extract
- ½ tsp. baking soda
- 1 tsp. Cream of tartar
- ¼ tsp. salt
- 1 tsp. ground cinnamon

Directions
1. Preheat the oven to 325 ° F.
2. Spray with a nonstick cooking spray on 2 baking sheets. In a large bowl, beat the unsalted butter and sugar until well combined.
3. Add the eggs, one at a time, bashing well after each one.
4. Whisk in the vanilla and the orange peel.
5. In a medium-size dish, combine the tartar cream, flour, baking soda, salt, and cinnamon.
6. To the butter mixture, add the dry ingredients and combine until blended.
7. Split the dough in two. Place each half on a sheet that has been prepared. Shape each half into a log form that is 3 inches wide and 3 quarters of an inch high with lightly floured hands. Bake for almost 35 min., till the dough logs, are smooth to the touch.
8. Remove the oven's dough logs and cool for 10 min.
9. Move logs to the surface of the work. Cut diagonally into ½-inch-thick slices utilizing serrated knives. On baking sheets, place cut side down.
10. Bake for almost 12 min. before the bottoms are golden.
11. Turn over the biscotti; bake for almost 12 min. more, till the bottoms are golden.
12. Before serving, switch to a rack and let it cool.

Nutrition Per Serving: Calories 149 Protein 2 g Sodium 76 mg Phosphorus 28 mg Fiber 0.5 g Potassium 53 mg

319.   APPLE CINNAMON FILLED PASTRIES

Preparation Time: 20 min.   **Cooking Time:** 15 min.   **Servings**: 6

Ingredients
- Apple mixture:
- ¼ cup of light brown sugar
- 4 apples
- ¼ cup unsalted butter, melted (for buttering the phyllo pastry sheets)
- 2 tbsp. unsalted butter, firm
- ¼ tsp. nutmeg
- 1 tsp. cinnamon
- 1 package phyllo dough (6 sheets)
- ¼ tsp. cornstarch
- 2 tbsp. vanilla extract
- Mix in a small bowl:
- 2 tbsp. cinnamon
- 3 tbsp. powdered sugar
- Optional: garnish with fresh mint sprigs, powdered sugar, and whipped cream

Directions
1. Apple mixture:
2. Preheat the oven to 350° F.
3. Sauté the apples in the butter for 6 to 8 min. in a wide sauté pan over medium-high flame.
4. Stir in the cinnamon, brown sugar, and nutmeg. Cook for 3 or 4 more min.
5. Mix the vanilla extract and cornstarch in a cup before it is dissolved. Stir in the apple mixture and simmer on a medium-high flame for an extra two min.
6. Turn off the heat and set aside the mixture.
7. Phyllo dough pastries:
8. Slightly grease a big 6-muffin tin pan.
9. Dust each side with the melted butter and then sprinkle with the cinnamon mix and powdered sugar, beginning with the phyllo dough's first sheet. Proceed till all 6 sheets of cinnamon mix

and sugar have been dusted and buttered, mounting one layer on top of the other as you go.

10. Slice the stack into 6 squares each. Using a stack of squares to line the sides and bottom of each muffin cup, leaving several of the squares dangling over the muffin cup's edges.

11. Fill with the apple mixture, each phyllo lined cup of muffin halfway to 3-quarters complete (this depends on how large the apples are

sliced), ensuring that every phyllo lined cup of the muffin has similar quantities of apple mixture.

12. In every muffin cup, fold the extra phyllo dough over apples.

13. Bake for 8 to 10 min. or till golden brown in the preheated oven at 350 ° F.

14. Optional: Garnish with fresh sprigs of mint, powdered sugar, or whipped cream.

Nutrition Per Serving: Calories 280 Protein 2 g Sodium 97 mg Phosphorus 33 mg Dietary Fiber 5 g Potassium 177 mg

320. SUNBURST LEMON BARS

Preparation Time: 1 h   **Cooking Time:** 45 min.   **Servings:**24

Ingredients

Crust:
- 1 cup unsalted butter (2 sticks), room temperature
- ½ cup sugar, powdered
- 2 cups flour, all-purpose

Filling:
- 1½ cups sugar
- 4 eggs
- ½ tsp. cream of tartar
- ¼ cup flour, all-purpose
- ¼ cup lemon juice
- ¼ tsp. baking soda

Glaze:
- 2 tbsp. lemon juice
- 1 cup sifted powdered sugar

Directions

Crust:
1. Preheat the oven to 350° F. Combine the powdered sugar, flour, and 1 cup of butter in a big bowl. Mix together till crumbly. In a 9" x 13" baking pan, push the mixture onto the bottom.
2. Bake for almost 15 to 20 min., till lightly browned.

Filling:
1. Beat the eggs gently in a medium-sized bowl.
2. Combine the flour, tartar cream, sugar, and baking soda in another bowl. In the eggs, add the dry mixture. Then to the egg mixture, add the lemon juice and mix till thickened slightly.
3. Pour it over the crust and bake for an additional 20 min. or till the filling is set.
4. Take it out of the oven and cool.

Glaze:
1. Mix the lemon juice steadily into the powdered sugar in a small bowl till it is spreadable. As desired, add less or more lemon juice.
2. Spread over the filling that has been cooled. Let the glaze settle and cut into 24 bars afterward. Hold the leftover lemon bars in the freezer.

Nutrition Per Serving: Calories 200 Protein 2 g Sodium 27 mg Phosphorus 32 mg Fiber 0.3 g Potassium 41 mg

321. GINGER- LEMON-COCONUT COOKIES

Preparation Time: 1 h   **Cooking Time:** 45 min.   **Servings:**12 cookies

Ingredients
- ½ cup sugar
- ½ cup butter (1 stick), unsalted
- ½ tsp. baking soda
- 1 egg
- 1 tbsp. lemon zest
- 1 cup unsweetened, toasted coconut
- 2 tbsp. lemon juice
- 1 ¼ cups flour
- 1 tbsp. chopped and peeled or grated, fresh ginger

Directions
1. Preheat the oven to 350° F.
2. Spread the unsweetened coconut on the baking sheet tray and bake for almost 5 to10 min. till the edges are light brown.
3. Take it out of the oven and put it aside in a bowl.
4. Cream the sugar and butter until fluffy and light using an electric mixer. Add the egg,

lemon juice, lemon zest and chopped ginger and blend until smooth.

5. Sift the flour and the baking soda together. In the butter mixture, stir the flour mixture and combine until fully mixed. For at least 30 min., cover and wait. Scoop out balls that are tbsp.-size and coil them in toasted coconut. Use a slightly lubricated baking sheet tray to put balls almost 2 inches apart.

6. Bake for 10 to12 min. till the edges are slightly brown. Remove and cool on a cool surface or counter.

Nutrition Per Serving: Calories 97 Protein 1 g Sodium 40 mg Phosphorus 17 mg Fiber 0.4 g Potassium 27 mg

322.   LEMON MOUSSE

Preparation time: 10 min. plus chill time.

Cooking time: 10 min.

Servings: 4

Ingredients:

- 1 cup coconut cream
- 8 ounces cream cheese, soft
- ¼ cup fresh lemon juice
- 3 pinches salt
- 1 tsp. lemon liquid stevia

Directions:

1. Preheat your oven to 350°F. Grease a ramekin with butter. Beat cream, cream cheese, fresh lemon juice, salt, and lemon liquid stevia in a mixer. Pour batter into ramekin.
2. Bake for 10 min., then transfer the mousse to a serving glass.
3. Let it chill for 2 hs and serve.
4. Enjoy!

Nutrition: Calories: 395 Fat: 31g Carbs: 3g Protein: 5g

323.   TART APPLE GRANITA

Preparation time: 15 min. 4 h freezing time.

Cooking time: 0

Servings: 4

Ingredients:

- ½ cup granulated sugar
- ½ cup water
- 2 cups unsweetened apple juice
- ¼ cup freshly squeezed lemon juice

Directions:

1. In a small saucepan over medium-high heat, heat the sugar and water.
2. Bring the mixture to a boil and then reduce the heat to low. Let it simmer for about 15 min. or until the liquid has reduced by half.
3. Remove the pan from the heat and pour the liquid into a large shallow metal pan.
4. Let the liquid cool for about 30 min., and then stir in the apple juice and lemon juice.
5. Place the pan in the freezer.
6. After 1 h, run a fork through the liquid to break up any ice crystals formed. Scrape down the sides as well.
7. Place the pan back in the freezer and repeat the stirring and scraping every 20 min., creating slush.
8. Serve when the mixture is completely frozen and looks like crushed ice, after about 3 hs.

Nutrition: Calories: 157 Fat: 0g Carbs: 0g Phosphorus: 10mg Potassium: 141mg Sodium: 5mg Protein: 0g

324.   RASPBERRY POPSICLE

Preparation time: 2 hs.

Cooking time: 15 min.

Servings: 4

Ingredients:

- 1 ½ cups raspberries
- 2 cups water

Directions:

1. Take a pan and fill it up with water.
2. Add raspberries.
3. Place it over medium heat and bring to water to a boil. Reduce the heat and simmer for 15 min.

4. Remove heat and pour the mix into Popsicle molds.

Nutrition: Calories: 58 Fat: 0.4g Carbs: 0g Protein: 1.4g

5. Add a Popsicle stick and let it chill for 2 hs.
6. Serve and enjoy!

325. EASY FUDGE

Preparation time: 15 min.   **Cooking time**: 5 min.   **Servings**: 25

Ingredients:

- 1 ¾ cups of coconut butter
- 1 cup pumpkin puree
- 1 tsp. ground cinnamon
- ¼ tsp. ground nutmeg
- 1 tbsp. coconut oil

Directions:

1. Take an 8x8 inch square baking pan and line it with aluminum foil. Take a spoon and scoop out the coconut butter into a heated pan and allow the butter to melt.
3. Keep stirring well and remove from the heat once fully melted.
4. Add spices and pumpkin and keep straining until you have a grain-like texture.
5. Add coconut oil and keep stirring to incorporate everything.
6. Scoop the mixture into your baking pan and evenly distribute it.
7. Place wax paper on top of the mixture and press gently to straighten the top.
8. Remove the paper and discard.
9. Allow it to chill for 1–2 hs.
10. Once chilled, take it out and slice it up into pieces.
11. Enjoy!

Nutrition: Calories: 120 Fat: 10g Carbs: 5g Protein: 1.2g

326. CRAMBERRY BAR

Preparation time: 35 min.   **Cooking time**: 25 min.   **Servings** 24 bars

Ingredients

Topping:

- 1 tsp. baking powder
- ½ cup flour, all-purpose
- ¾ cup of sugar
- 1 cup cranberries, dried
- 1 tsp. vanilla extract
- 4 eggs, large
- Optional: Powdered sugar (for dusting)

Crust:

- 1 1/3 cups of sugar
- 1 ½ cups flour, all-purpose
- ¾ cup butter (1 1/2 sticks), unsalted

Directions

1. Preheat the oven to 350° F.
2. Stir together the flour and sugar in a medium-sized bowl; slice in unsalted butter till the mixture holds together. Pat into the 9" x 13" ungreased baking pan. Bake till slightly browned, for 10 min.
3. In a small bowl, sift the baking powder and flour together to prepare the topping. Put the dried cranberries in. Set aside.
4. Mix the sugar, vanilla, and eggs in a medium-size bowl. Add a mixture of flour. Add onto baked crust. For 20 to 25 min., bake.
5. While warm, cut into 24 bars and brush with powdered sugar.

Nutrition Per Serving: Calories 190 Protein 2 g Sodium 34 mg Phosphorus 34 mg Fiber 0.6 g Potassium 28 mg

327. MOLTEN CHOCOLATE MINT BROWNIES

Preparation time: 40 min.   **Cooking time**:30 min.   **Servings**: 12 brownies

Ingredients

1. 1 box of Betty Crocker brownie mix, not supreme
2. 12 Andes chocolates, mint

3. Optional garnish: cocoa powder (sweetened or unsweetened), powdered sugar, fresh mint sprigs

Directions

1. Preheat the oven and ready the mixture of brownie according to the box's instructions.
2. Prepare a lining or finely greased 12 cup muffin tin and flour the sides and bottom. Pour the brownie mixture onto the pan and bake for 25 min. Take the brownies out of the oven and place one bit of mint candy in the middle and bake for an extra 5 min. Turn the oven off and take it. For 5–10 min., let cool.
3. Take the brownie cupcakes out of the pan, then serve.
4. Optional: Dust with powdered sugar and cocoa powder and garnish with the fresh mint

Nutrition Per Serving: Calories 307 Protein 3 g Sodium 147 mg Phosphorus 61 mg Fiber 0 g Potassium 120 mg

328. CREAM CHEESE SUGAR COOKIES

Preparation time: 10 min.   **Cooking time**: 10 min.   **Servings** 48 servings

Ingredients

- 1 cup softened, unsalted butter
- 1 cup of sugar
- 1 egg, large, separated
- 3 oz. softened cream cheese
- ¼ tsp. almond extract
- ½ tsp. salt
- 2¼ cups flour, all-purpose
- ½ tsp. vanilla extract
- Optional: garnish with colored sugar

Directions

1. Place the butter, sugar, cream cheese, almond extract, salt, egg yolk, and vanilla extract in a large bowl. Blend thoroughly. Stir in the flour till it is well-mixed.
2. Chill the cookie dough in the fridge for 2 hs.
3. Preheat the oven to 350° F.
4. Roll out the pastry, one third at a time to ¼-inch width, on a thinly floured board. Break using thinly floured cookie cutters into ideal forms.
5. Place them on ungreased cookie sheets 1 inch apart. Dust with egg white, which is slightly beaten and sprinkle with the colored sugar or leave the cookies plain if desired.
6. For 7 to 9 min. or till light golden brown, bake the cream cheese cookies. Before serving, let it cool completely.

Nutrition Per Serving: Calories 79 Protein 1 g Sodium 33 mg Phosphorus 11 mg Fiber 0 g Potassium 11 mg

329. ICE CREAM PUMPKIN PIE

Preparation time: 10 min.   **Cooking time**:0 min.   **Servings** 8

Ingredients

- 1 cup pumpkin, canned
- 1 pint or 2 cups softened vanilla ice cream.
- 1/2 tsp. ginger
- 3/4 cup of sugar
- 1/4 tsp. nutmeg
- 1/2 tsp. cinnamon
- 1 9" baked pie shell
- 1 cup whipped topping

Directions

1. Mix all the ingredients in the food processor, except the pie shell, till well mixed.
2. Pour the mixture into the baked pie shell and freeze till firm.

Nutrition Per Serving: Calories 275 Protein 3 g Sodium 118 mg Phosphorus 51 mg Potassium 90 mg

330. SWEET CHERRY COBBLER

Preparation time: 55 min.   **Cooking time**: 40 min.   **Servings** 12

Ingredients

Cherry Filling

- 2/3 cup sugar, granulated
- 5 cups halved and pitted red cherries, sweet, about 1.7 lbs.
- 1/4 tsp. salt
- 1/4 tsp. almond extract
- 2 tbsp. cornstarch
- 1 tsp. vanilla extract
- 2 tbsp. lemon juice

Cobbler Topping

- 1/2 cup sugar
- 1 cup flour, all-purpose
- 1/2 cup cold milk, non-fat
- 1/4 tsp. salt
- 1 tsp. baking powder
- 2 tbsp. unsalted, cubed, and cold butter
- 1/4 tsp. ground cinnamon

Directions

1. Preheat your oven to 450°F.
2. Cherry Filling
3. Prepare the cherries. To pit the cherries, you may split the cherries in two, either remove the pits or use a solid straw-like one with a reusable plastic cup. Force the straw up from the bottom of the cherry through the tip. The pit's going to pop straight out. Cut the cherries from the middle, then. This procedure is a little sloppy but preparing the cherries in half can reduce the time.
4. In a big saucepan, put the sugar, cherries, salt, cornstarch, and whisk in the lemon juice, almond extract and vanilla extract.
5. Carry to a boil on medium flame and cook for around 5 to 7 min. till the cherries are tenderized and the juices are thickened.
6. Pour the filling of the cherry into an ungreased baking pan of 8-inches. (Round or square.)
7. Cobbler Topping
8. In a medium bowl, put the sugar, flour, baking powder, cinnamon, and salt and stir until combined.
9. Slice in the butter using a pastry blender or fork, so the mixture looks like coarse crumbs.
10. In limited quantities, add the milk slowly, only enough to lubricate the dough. (Maybe you might not need all the milk.)
11. Drop the spoonful of dough on the top of the filling a cookie dough scoop or a soup spoon. Leave several airflow gaps such that between the scoops of the dough, the filling will bubble up. Bake till the top is golden brown, for 10 to 15 min. Using a toothpick, test for doneness. Upon thoroughly cooking the dough topping, the toothpick must be clean.
12. Serve warm, or up to 1 week you can keep in the fridge. To Reheat, let it stand for at least 30 min. to one h at room temperature and reheat for 10 to 15 min. at 350 °F.

Nutrition Per Serving: Calories 117 Protein 2 g Sodium 103 mg Phosphorus 65 mg Fiber 2 g Potassium 186 mg

331.   MINI PINEAPPLE CAKE

Preparation time: 50 min.   **Cooking time**: 40 min.   **Servings** 12

Ingredients

- 1/3 cup brown sugar, packed
- 3 tbsp. melted butter, unsalted
- 6 cherries, sliced into halves, fresh and pitted
- 12 canned pineapple slices, unsweetened
- 2/3 cup milk, fat-free
- 1/4 tsp. salt
- 2/3 cup sugar
- 1 egg
- 3 tbsp. canola oil
- 1/2 tsp. vanilla extract
- 1 tsp. lemon juice
- 1-1/4 tsp. baking powder
- 1-1/3 cups of cake flour

Directions

1. Pour batter into a muffin pan with 12 servings. Square pan for baking.
2. Sprinkle each segment with a little bit of brown sugar.
3. Press one slice of pineapple into each segment to create a cup shape. In the middle of each pineapple slice, put one half of the cherry (cut side must be facing up) and set aside.
4. Beat the oil, milk, sugar, egg and extracts in a wide bowl until well mixed. Combine the baking powder, salt, and flour; beat into the sugar mixture till mixed. In a muffin pan, mix into the prepared batter.
5. For 35 to 40 min., bake at 350°F or till a toothpick comes out clean. Invert the muffin pan directly and transfer the cooked cakes into a serving tray. If required, you may use a butter knife or a tiny spatula around the edges to gently extract them from the pan. Serve it warm.

Nutrition Per Serving: Calories 193 Protein 3 g Sodium 131 mg Phosphorus 88 mg Fiber 1 g Potassium 169 mg

332.   PUMPKIN CHEESECAKE

Preparation time: 10 min.   **Cooking time**: 50 min.   **Servings**: 4

Ingredients:

- 2 ½ tbsp. unsalted butter
- 4-ounces cream cheese
- ½ cup all-purpose white flour
- 3 tbsp. golden brown sugar
- ¼ cup granulated sugar
- ½ cup pureed pumpkin
- 2 egg whites
- 1 tsp. ground cinnamon
- 1 tsp. ground nutmeg
- 1 tsp. vanilla extract

Directions:
1. Preheat the oven to 350°F.
2. Mix brown sugar and flour in a container.
3. Mix in the butter to form 'breadcrumbs.'
4. Place ¾ of this mixture in a dish.
5. Bake in the oven for 15 min. Remove and cool. Lightly whisk the egg and fold in the cream cheese, sugar, pumpkin, cinnamon, nutmeg, and vanilla until smooth.
6. Pour this mixture over the oven-baked base and sprinkle with the rest of the breadcrumbs from earlier. Bake for 30 to 35 min. more.
7. Cool, slice, and serve.

Nutrition: Calories: 248 Fat: 13g Carb: 33g Phosphorus: 67mg Potassium: 96mg Sodium: 146mg Protein: 4g

333. COCONUT LOAF

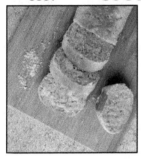

Preparation time: 15 min.
Cooking time: 40 min.
Servings: 4
Ingredients:
- 1 ½ tbsp. coconut flour
- ¼ tsp. baking powder
- 1/8 tsp. salt
- 1 tbsp. coconut oil, melted
- 1 whole egg

Directions:
1. Preheat your oven to 350°F.
2. Add coconut flour, baking powder, salt.
3. Add coconut oil, eggs and stir well until mixed.
4. Leave the batter for several min.
5. Pour half the batter onto the baking pan.
6. Spread it to form a circle, repeat with the remaining batter. Bake in the oven for 10 min.
7. Once a golden-brown texture comes, let it cool and serve. Enjoy!

Nutrition: Calories: 297 Fat: 14g Carbs: 15g Protein: 15g

334. CHOCOLATE PARFAIT

Preparation time: 2 hs.   **Cooking time**: 0 min.   **Servings**: 4
Ingredients:
- 2 tbsp. cocoa powder
- 1 cup almond milk
- 1 tbsp. chia seeds
- Pinch of salt
- ½ tsp. vanilla extract

Directions:
1. Take a bowl and add cocoa powder, almond milk, chia seeds, vanilla extract, pinch of salt and stir.
2. Transfer to dessert glass and place in your fridge for 2 hs.
3. Serve and enjoy!

Nutrition: Calories: 130 Fat: 5g Carbs: 7g Protein: 16g

335. VANILLA CUSTARD

Preparation time: 7 min.   **Cooking time**: 10 min.   **Servings:** 10
Ingredients:
- 1 egg
- 1/8 tsp. vanilla
- 1/8 tsp. nutmeg
- ½ cup almond milk
- 2 tbsp. stevia

Directions:
1. Scald the milk, then let it cool a little.
2. Break the egg into a bowl and beat it with the nutmeg.
3. Add the scalded milk, the vanilla, and the sweetener to taste. Mix well.

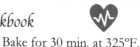
4 Place the bowl in a baking pan filled with ½ deep of water.
5 Bake for 30 min. at 325°F.
6 Serve.

Nutrition: Calories: 167.3 Fat: 9g Carb: 11g Phosphorus: 205mg Potassium: 249mg Sodium: 124mg Protein: 10g

336.   ALMOND CRACKERS

Preparation time: 10 min.   **Cooking time**: 20 min.   **Servings**: 40 crackers.

Ingredients:
- 1 cup almond flour
- ¼ tsp. baking soda
- ¼ tsp. salt
- 1/8 tsp. black pepper
- 3 tbsp. sesame seeds
- 1 egg, beaten
- Salt and pepper to taste

Directions:
1 Pre-heat your oven to 350°F.
2 Line two baking sheets with parchment paper and keep them on the side.
3 Mix the dry ingredients into a large bowl and add egg, mix well and form a dough. Divide dough into two balls. Roll out the dough between two pieces of parchment paper.
4 Cut into crackers and transfer them to prepare a baking sheet.
5 Bake for 15–20 min.
6 Repeat until all the dough has been used up.
7 Leave crackers to cool and serve.
8 Enjoy!

Nutrition: Calories: 302 Fat: 28g Carbs: 4g Protein: 9g

337.   LEMON THINS

Preparation Time: 15 min   **Cooking Time**: 8 to 10 min   **Servings**: 30 cookies

Ingredients:
- Cooking spray
- 11/4 cups whole wheat pastry flour
- 1/3 cup cornstarch
- 11/2 tsp. baking powder
- ¾ cup sugar, divided
- 2 tbsp. butter, softened
- 2 tbsp. extra-virgin olive oil
- 1 large egg white
- 3 tsp. freshly grated lemon zest
- 11/2 tsp. vanilla extract
- 4 tbsp. freshly squeezed lemon juice

Directions:
1. Preheat the oven to 350°F. Coat two baking sheets with cooking spray. In a mixing bowl, whisk together the flour, cornstarch, and baking powder. In another mixing bowl beat 1/2 cup of the sugar, the butter, and olive oil with an electric mixer on medium speed until fluffy.
2. Add the egg white, lemon zest, and vanilla and beat until smooth. Beat in the lemon juice.
3. Add the dry ingredients to the wet ingredients and fold in with a rubber spatula just until combined.
4. Drop the dough by the tsp.ful, 2 inches apart, onto the prepared baking sheets.
5. Place the remaining 1/4 cup sugar in a saucer. Coat the bottom of a wide-bottomed glass with cooking spray and dip it in the sugar. Flatten the dough with the glass bottom into 21/2-inch circles, dipping the glass in the sugar each time.
6. Bake the cookies until they are just starting to brown around the edges, 8 to 10 min. Transfer to a flat surface (not a rack) to crisp.

Nutrition: (1 cookie) Calories: 40; Total Fat 2g; Saturated Fat: 1g; Cholesterol: 2mg; Sodium: 26mg; Potassium: 3mg; Total Carbs: 5g; Fiber: 1g; Protein: 1g

338.   SNICKERDOODLE CHICKPEA BLONDIES

Preparation Time: 10 min   **Cooking Time**: 30 to 35 min   **Servings**: 15

Ingredients:
- 1 (15-ounce) can chickpeas, drained and rinsed
- 3 tbsp. nut butter of choice
- ¾ tsp. baking powder
- 2 tsp. vanilla extract
- 1/8 tsp. baking soda
- ¾ cup brown sugar
- 1 tbsp. unsweetened applesauce
- 1/4 cup ground flaxseed meal

↪ 21/4 tsp. cinnamon

Directions:

1. Preheat the oven to 350°F. Grease an 8-by-8-inch baking pan. Blend all ingredients in a food processor until very smooth. Scoop into the prepared baking pan.

2. Bake until the tops are medium golden brown, 30 to 35 min. Allow the brownies to cool completely before cutting.

Nutrition: Calories: 85; Total Fat 2g; Saturated Fat: 0g; Cholesterol: 0mg; Sodium: 7mg; Potassium: 62mg; Total Carbs: 16g; Fiber: 2g; Protein: 3g

339. CHOCOLATE CHIA SEED PUDDING

Preparation Time: 15 min   **Cooking Time**: 0 min   **Servings**: 4

Ingredients:

↪ 11/2 cups unsweetened vanilla almond milk
↪ 1/4 cup unsweetened cocoa powder
↪ 1/4 cup maple syrup (or substitute any sweetener)
↪ 1/2 tsp. vanilla extract
↪ 1/3 cup chia seeds
↪ 1/2 cup strawberries
↪ 1/4 cup blueberries
↪ 1/4 cup raspberries
↪ 2 tbsp. unsweetened coconut flakes
↪ 1/4 to 1/2 tsp. ground cinnamon (optional)

Directions:

1. Add the almond milk, cocoa powder, maple syrup, and vanilla extract to a blender and blend until smooth. Whisk in chia seeds.

2. In a small bowl, gently mash the strawberries with a fork. Distribute the strawberry mash evenly to the bottom of 4 glass jars.

3. Pour equal portions of the blended milk-cocoa mixture into each of the jars and let the pudding rest in the refrigerator until it achieves a pudding like consistency, at least 3 to 5 hours and up to overnight.

Nutrition: Calories: 189; Total Fat 7g; Saturated Fat: 2g; Cholesterol: 0mg; Sodium: 60mg; Potassium: 232mg; Total Carbs: 28g; Fiber: 10g; Protein: 6g

340. CHOCOLATE-MINT TRUFFLES

Preparation Time: 45 min   **Cooking Time**: 5 hours   **Servings**: 60 small truffles

Ingredients:

↪ 14 ounces semisweet chocolate, coarsely chopped
↪ ¾ cup half-and-half
↪ 1/2 tsp. pure vanilla extract
↪ 11/2 tsp. peppermint extract
↪ 2 tbsp. unsalted butter, softened
↪ ¾ cup naturally unsweetened or Dutch-process cocoa powder

Directions:

1. Place semisweet chocolate in a large heatproof bowl. Microwave in four 15-second increments, stirring after each, for a total of 60 seconds. Stir until almost completely melted. Set aside. In a small saucepan over medium heat, heat the half-and-half, whisking occasionally, until it just begins to boil. Remove from the heat, then whisk in the vanilla and peppermint extracts.

2. Pour the mixture over the chocolate and, using a wooden spoon, gently stir in one direction.

3. Once the chocolate and cream are smooth, stir in the butter until it is combined and melted.

4. Cover with plastic wrap pressed on the top of the mixture, and then let it sit at room temperature for 30 min.

5. After 30 min, place the mixture in the refrigerator until it is thick and can hold a ball shape, about 5 hours.

6. Line a large baking sheet with parchment paper or a use a silicone baking mat. Set aside.

7. Remove the mixture from the refrigerator. Place the cocoa powder in a bowl.

8. Scoop 1 tsp. of the ganache and, using your hands, roll into a ball. Roll the ball in the cocoa powder, the place on the prepared baking sheet. (You can coat your palms with a little cocoa powder to prevent sticking).

9. Serve immediately or cover and store at room temperature for up to 1 week.

Nutrition: Calories: 21; Total Fat 2g; Saturated Fat: 1g; Cholesterol: 2mg; Sodium: 2mg; Potassium: 21mg; Total Carbs: 2g; Fiber: 1g; Protein: 0g

341.   PERSONAL MANGO PIES

Preparation Time: 15 min   **Cooking Time**: 14 to 16 min   **Servings**: 12

Ingredients:

- Cooking spray
- 12 small wonton wrappers
- 1 tbsp. cornstarch
- 1/2 cup water
- 3 cups finely chopped mango (fresh, or thawed from frozen, no sugar added)
- 2 tbsp. brown sugar (not packed)
- 1/2 tsp. cinnamon
- 1 tbsp. light whipped butter or buttery spread

Directions:

1. Unsweetened coconut flakes (optional)
2. Preheat the oven to 350°F.
3. Spray a 12-cup muffin pan with nonstick cooking spray. Place a wonton wrapper into each cup of the muffin pan, pressing it into the bottom and up along the sides.
4. Lightly spray the wrappers with nonstick spray. Bake until lightly browned, about 8 min.
5. Meanwhile, in a medium nonstick saucepan, combine the cornstarch with the water and stir

to dissolve. Add the mango, brown sugar, and cinnamon and turn heat to medium.

6. Stirring frequently, cook until the mangoes have slightly softened and the mixture is thick and gooey, 6 to 8 min.
7. Remove the mango mixture from heat and stir in the butter.
8. Spoon the mango mixture into wonton cups, about 3 tbsp. each. Top with coconut flakes (if using) and serve warm.

Nutrition: Calories: 61; Total Fat 1g; Saturated Fat: 0g; Cholesterol: 2mg; Sodium: 52mg; Potassium: 77mg; Total Carbs: 14g; Fiber: 1g; Protein: 1g

342.   GRILLED PEACH SUNDAES

Preparation Time: 15 min   **Cooking Time**: 5 min   **Servings**: 1

Ingredients:

- 1 tbsp. toasted unsweetened coconut
- 1 tsp. canola oil
- 2 peaches, halved and pitted
- 2 scoops non-fat vanilla yogurt, frozen

Directions:

1. Brush the peaches with oil and grill until tender.
2. Place peach halves on a bowl and top with frozen yogurt and coconut.

Nutrition: Calories: 61; Carbs: 2g; Protein: 2g; Fats: 6g; Phosphorus: 32mg; Potassium: 85mg; Sodium: 30mg

343.   BLUEBERRY CAKE

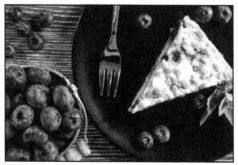

Preparation Time: 15 min
Cooking Time: 45 min
Servings: 9
Ingredients:
- 1/2 cup margarine
- 1 1/4 cups reduced fat milk
- 1 cup granulated sugar
- 1 egg
- 1 egg white
- 1 tbsp. lemon zest, grated
- 1 tsp. cinnamon
- 1/3 cup light brown sugar

- 2 1/2 cups fresh blueberries
- 2 1/2 cups self-rising flour

Directions:

1. Cream the margarine and granulated sugar using an electric mixer at high speed until fluffy. Add the egg and egg white and beat for another two min. Add the lemon zest and reduce the speed to low.
2. Add the flour with milk alternately.
3. In a greased 13x19 pan, spread half of the batter and sprinkle with blueberry on top. Add the remaining batter. Bake in a 350-degree Fahrenheit preheated oven for 45 min.
4. Let it cool on a wire rack before slicing and serving.

Nutrition: Calories: 384; Carbs: 63g; Protein: 7g; Fats: 13g; Phosphorus: 264mg; Potassium: 158mg; Sodium: 456mg

344.   FESTIVE BERRY PARFAIT

Preparation time: 1 h 20 min.   **Cooking time**: 0 min.   **Servings**: 4

Ingredients:

- 1 cup vanilla rice milk, at room temperature
- ½ cup plain cream cheese, at room temperature
- 1 tbsp. granulated sugar
- ½ tsp. ground cinnamon
- 1 cup crumbled Meringue Cookies (here)
- 2 cups fresh blueberries
- 1 cup sliced fresh strawberries

Directions:

1. Whisk together the milk, cream cheese, sugar, and cinnamon until smooth in a small bowl,
2. Into 4 (6-ounce) glasses, spoon ¼ cup of crumbled cookie in the bottom of each. Spoon ¼ cup of the cream cheese mixture on top of the cookies.
3. Top the cream cheese with ¼ cup of the berries.
4. Repeat in each cup with the cookies, cream cheese mixture, and berries.
5. Chill in the refrigerator for 1 hour and serve.

Nutrition: Calories: 243kcal Fat: 11g Carbs: 33g Phosphorus: 84mg Potassium: 189mg Sodium: 145mg Protein: 4g

345.   CHORIZO AND EGG TORTILLA

Preparation time: 10 min.   **Cooking time**: 13 min.   **Servings**: 1 tortilla

Ingredients:

- 1 flour tortilla, about 6-inches
- 1/3 cup chorizo meat, chopped
- 1 egg

Directions:

1. Take a medium-sized skillet pan, place it over medium heat.
2. When it is hot, add chorizo and cook for 5 to 8 min until done.
3. When the meat has cooked, drain the excess fat, whisk an egg, pour it into the pan, stir until combined, and cook for 3 min, or until eggs have cooked. Spoon egg onto the tortilla and then serve.

Nutrition: Calories: 223 Cholesterol: 211ml Fat: 11g Net Carbs: 13.5g Protein: 16g Sodium: 317mg Carbs: 15g Phosphorus: 232mg Fiber: 1.5g

346.   CORN PUDDING

Preparation time: 10 min.   **Cooking time**: 40 min.   **Servings**: 6

Ingredients:

- Unsalted butter, for greasing the baking dish
- 2 tbsp. all-purpose flour
- ½ tsp. Ener-G baking soda substitute
- 3 eggs
- ¾ cup unsweetened rice milk, at room temperature
- 3 tbsp. unsalted butter, melted
- 2 tbsp. light sour cream
- 2 tbsp. granulated sugar
- 2 cups frozen corn kernels, thawed

Directions:

1. Preheat the oven to 350°F.

2. Somehow grease an 8-by-8-inch baking dish with butter; set aside.
3. In a small bowl, mix the flour and baking soda substitute; set aside.
4. In a medium bowl, whisk together the eggs, rice milk, butter, sour cream, and sugar.
5. Stir the flour mixture into the egg mixture until smooth. Add the corn to the batter and stir until very well mixed.
6. Spoon the batter into the baking dish and bake for about 40 min or until the pudding is set.
7. Let the pudding cool for about 15 min and serve warm.

Nutrition: Calories: 175 Fat: 10g Carbs: 19g Phosphorus: 111mg Potassium: 170mg Sodium: 62mg Protein: 5g

347.   RHUBARB BREAD PUDDING

Preparation time: 15 min.   **Cooking time**: 50 min.   **Servings**: 6

Ingredients:
- Unsalted butter
- 3 eggs
- 1½ cups unsweetened rice milk
- ½ cup granulated sugar
- 1 tbsp. cornstarch
- 1 vanilla bean, split
- 10 thick pieces of white bread
- 2 cups chopped fresh rhubarb

Directions:
1 Preheat the oven to 350°F.
2 In a bowl, whisk the eggs, sugar, rice milk, and cornstarch.
3 Scrape the vanilla seeds into the milk mixture and whisk to blend.
4 Place the bread in the egg combination and stir to coat the bread totally.
5 Add the chopped rhubarb and stir to combine.
6 Allow the bread and egg mixture to be the marinade for 30 min.
7 Spoon the combination, put it in the arranged baking dish, conceal it with aluminum foil, and then bake for 40 min.
8 Bare the bread pudding, then bake for an extra 10 min or up until the pudding is golden brown and set. Serve the dish warm.

Dialysis modification: Decrease the rhubarb to 1 cup to bring the potassium to less than 150mg per serving. Or omit the rhubarb completely to bring the potassium to less than 75mg per serving. The bread pudding is delicious without the rhubarb, but it will be less tart.

Nutrition: Calories: 197kcal Fat: 4g Carbs: 35g Phosphorus: 109mg Potassium: 192mg Sodium: 159mg Protein: 6g

348.   FRUIT AND CHEESE WRAP

Preparation time: 10 min.   **Cooking time**: 0 min.   **Servings**: 2

Ingredients:
- 2 (6-inch) flour tortillas
- 2 tbsp. plain cream cheese
- 1 apple, peeled, cored, and sliced thin
- 1 tbsp. honcy

Directions:
1 Place both tortillas on a clean work surface and spread 1 tbsp. of cream cheese onto each tortilla, leaving about ½ inch around the edges.
2 Arrange the apple slices on the cream cheese, just in the center of the tortilla on the side closest to you, leaving about 1½ inches on each side and 2 inches on the bottom.
3 Drizzle the apples lightly with honey.
4 Fold the tortillas' left and right edges into the center, placing the edge over the apples.
5 Taking the tortilla edge closest to you, fold it over the fruit and the side pieces. Roll the tortilla away from you, creating a snug wrap. Repeat with the second tortilla.

Nutrition: Calories: 188kcal Fat: 6g Carbs: 33g Phosphorus: 73mg Potassium: 136mg Sodium: 177mg Protein: 4g

349.   EGG-IN-THE-HOLE

Preparation time: 5 min.   **Cooking time**: 5 min.   **Servings**: 2

Ingredients:
- (½-inch-thick) slices Italian bread
- ¼ cup unsalted butter
- eggs
- 2 tbsp. chopped fresh chives
- Pinch cayenne pepper
- Freshly ground black pepper

Directions:

1. Make use of a cookie cutter or a small glass, slice a 2-inch round from the center of each piece of bread.
2. Using a large nonstick skillet over medium-high heat, thaw the butter.
3. Place the bread in the skillet, toast it for 1 min, and then flip the bread.
4. Open the eggs into the holes in the center of the bread, then cooks for about 2 min. You may wait until the eggs are set, and the bread is golden brown.Top with chopped chives, cayenne pepper, and black pepper.
5. Cook the bread for additional 2 min.
6. Transfer an egg-in-the-hole to each plate to serve.

Nutrition: Calories: 304kcal Fat: 29g Carbs: 12g Phosphorus: 119mg Potassium: 109mg Sodium: 204mg Protein: 9g

350.   SKILLET-BAKED PANCAKE

Preparation time: 15 min.

Cooking time: 20 min.

Servings: 2

Ingredients:

- 2 eggs
- ½ cup unsweetened rice milk
- ½ cup all-purpose flour
- ¼ tsp. ground cinnamon
- Pinch ground nutmeg
- Cooking spray, for greasing the skillet

Directions:

1. Pre-heat the oven to 450°F.
2. In a medium container, mix the eggs and rice milk.
3. Stir in the cinnamon, flour, and nutmeg up until it is blended. Make sure it is still slightly bumpy, but do not overmix. Then spray a 9-inch ovenproof frying pan thru cooking spray and place the skillet in the pre-heated oven for 5 min.
4. Take away the skillet cautiously and pour the pancake batter into the skillet.
5. Put back the skillet to the oven.
6. Bake the pancake for around 20 min. You may wait until it is puffed up and crispy on the edges.
7. Slice the pancake into halves, then serve.

Dialysis modification: If you need additional protein in this dish, whisk in an extra egg white. There will be no change in texture or taste.

Nutrition: Calories: 161kcal Fat: 1g Carbs: 30g Phosphorus: 73mg Potassium: 106mg Sodium: 79mg Protein: 7g

351.   PEANUT BUTTER COOKIES

Preparation Time: 15 min   **Cooking Time**: 24 min   **Servings**: 24

Ingredients:

- 1/4 cup granulated sugar
- 1 cup unsalted peanut butter
- 1 tsp. baking soda
- 2 cups all-purpose flour
- 2 large eggs
- 2 tbsp. butter
- 2 tsp. pure vanilla extract
- 4 ounces softened cream cheese

Directions:

1. Line a cookie sheet with a non-stick liner. Set aside.
2. In a bowl, mix flour, sugar and baking soda. Set aside.
3. On a mixing bowl, combine the butter, cream cheese and peanut butter.
4. Mix on high speed until it forms a smooth consistency. Add the eggs and vanilla gradually while mixing until it forms a smooth consistency.
5. Add the almond flour mixture slowly and mix until well combined.
6. The dough is ready once it starts to stick together into a ball.
7. Scoop the dough using a 1 tbsp. cookie scoop and drop each cookie on the prepared cookie sheet.
8. Press the cookie with a fork and bake for 10 to 12 min at 350 F.

Nutrition: Calories: 138; Carbs: 12g; Protein: 4g; Fats: 9g; Phosphorus: 60mg; Potassium: 84mg; Sodium: 31mg

352.   GOOD SCONES

Preparation Time: 15 min   **Cooking Time**: 12 min   **Servings**: 10

Ingredients:

- ⚐ 1/4 cup dried cranberries
- ⚐ 1/4 cup sunflower seeds
- ⚐ 1/2 tsp. baking soda
- ⚐ 1 large egg
- ⚐ cups all-purpose flour
- ⚐ tbsp. honey

Directions:

1. Preheat the oven to 3500F.
2. Grease a baking sheet. Set aside.
3. In a bowl, mix the salt, baking soda and flour. Add the dried fruits, nuts and seeds. Set aside.
4. In another bowl, mix the honey and eggs.
5. Add the wet ingredients to the dry ingredients. Use your hands to mix the dough.
6. Create 10 small round dough and place them on the baking sheet.
7. Bake for 12 min.

Nutrition: Calories: 44; carbs: 27g; protein: 4g; fats: 3g; phosphorus: 59mg; potassium: 92mg; sodium: 65mg

353. MIXED BERRY COBBLER

Preparation Time: 15 min   **Cooking Time**: 4 hours   **Servings**: 8

Ingredients:

- ⚐ 1/4 cup coconut milk
- ⚐ 1/4 cup ghee
- ⚐ 1/4 cup honey
- ⚐ 1/2 cup almond flour
- ⚐ 1/2 cup tapioca starch
- ⚐ 1/2 tbsp. cinnamon
- ⚐ 1/2 tbsp. coconut sugar
- ⚐ 1 tsp. vanilla
- ⚐ 12 ounces frozen raspberries
- ⚐ 16 ounces frozen wild blueberries
- ⚐ 2 tsp. baking powder
- ⚐ 2 tsp. tapioca starch

Directions:

1. Place the frozen berries in the slow cooker. Add honey and 2 tsp. of tapioca starch. Mix to combine. In a bowl, mix the tapioca starch, almond flour, coconut milk, ghee, baking powder and vanilla. Sweeten with sugar. Place this pastry mix on top of the berries.
2. Set the slow cooker for 4 hours.

Nutrition: Calories: 146; Carbs: 33g; Protein: 1g; Fats: 3g; Phosphorus: 29mg; Potassium: 133mg; Sodium: 4mg

28-DAY MEAL PLAN

DAY	BREAKFAST	LUNCH	DINNER	DESSERTS
1	Breakfast Salad from Grains and Fruits	Saucy Garlic Greens	Eggplant and Red Pepper Soup	Chocolate Trifle
2	French toast with Applesauce	Garden Salad	Seafood Casserole	Pineapple Meringues
3	Bagels Made Healthy	Spicy Cabbage Dish	Ground Beef and Rice Soup	Baked Custard
4	Cornbread with Southern Twist	Extreme Balsamic Chicken	Couscous Burgers	Strawberry Pie
5	Grandma's Pancake Special	Enjoyable Spinach and Bean Medley	Baked Flounder	Apple Crisp
6	Very Berry Smoothie	Tantalizing Cauliflower and Dill Mash	Persian Chicken	Almond Cookies
7	Pasta with Indian Lentils	Secret Asian Green Beans	Pork Souvlaki	Lime Pie
8	Apple Pumpkin Muffins	Excellent Acorn Mix	Pork Meatloaf	Buttery Lemon Squares
9	Spiced French Toast	Crunchy Almond Chocolate Bars	Chicken Stew	Blackberry Cream Cheese Pie
10	Breakfast Tacos	Golden Eggplant Fries	Beef Chili	Apple Cinnamon Pie
11	Mexican Scrambled Eggs in Tortilla	Lettuce and Chicken Platter	Shrimp Paella	Maple Crisp Bars
12	American Blueberry Pancakes	Greek Lemon Chicken Bowl	Salmon & Pesto Salad	Pineapple Gelatin Pie
13	Raspberry Peach Breakfast Smoothie	Spicy Chili Crackers	Baked Fennel & Garlic Sea Bass	Chocolate Gelatin Mousse
14	Fast Microwave Egg Scramble	Dolmas Wrap	Lemon, Garlic & Cilantro Tuna and Rice	Cheesecake Bites
15	Mango Lassi Smoothie	Green Palak Paneer	Cod & Green Bean Risotto	Pumpkin Bites
16	Breakfast Maple Sausage	Sporty Baby Carrots	Sardine Fish Cakes	Protein Balls
17	Summer Veggie Omelet	Traditional Black Bean Chili	Cajun Catfish	Cashew Cheese Bites
18	Raspberry Overnight Porridge	Very Wild Mushroom Pilaf	4-Ingredients Salmon Fillet	Healthy Cinnamon Lemon Tea
19	Cheesy Scrambled Eggs with Fresh Herbs	Chilled Chicken, Artichoke and Zucchini Platter	Spanish Cod in Sauce	Mint Ginger Tea

20	Turkey and Spinach Scramble on Melba Toast	Chicken and Carrot Stew	Fish Shakshuka	Energy Booster Sunflower Balls
21	Vegetable Omelet	Tasty Spinach Pie	Eggplant and Red Pepper Soup	Simple Berry Sorbet
22	Mixed Vegetable Barley	Tuna Twist	Parsley Scallops	Rhubarb Bread Pudding
23	Spicy Sesame Tofu	Ciabatta Rolls with Chicken Pesto	Blackened Chicken	Fruit and Cheese Wrap
24	Mushroom Rice Noodles	Marinated Shrimp Pasta Salad	Spicy Paprika Lamb Chops	Egg-In-The-Hole
25	Egg Fried Rice	Peanut Butter and Jelly Grilled Sandwich	Mushroom and Olive Steak	Skillet-Baked Pancake
26	Vegetable Rice Casserole	Grilled Onion and Cheese Sandwich	Parsley and Chicken Breast	Peanut Butter Cookies
27	French Toast Special	Crispy Lemon Chicken	Apple-Chai Smoothie	Mixed Berry Cobbler
28	Turkey Scramble on Toast	Chicken Egg Rolls	Watermelon-Raspberry Smoothie	Good Scones

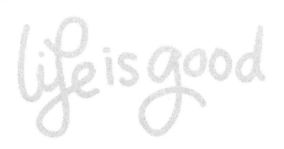

CONCLUSION

You likely had little knowledge about your kidneys before. You probably didn't know how you could take steps to improve your kidney health and decrease the risk of developing kidney failure. However, through reading this book, you now understand the power of the human kidney and chronic kidney disease prognosis. While over thirty-million Americans are being affected by kidney disease, you can now take steps to be one of the people who is actively working to promote your kidney health. Kidney disease currently ranks as the 18th deadliest condition in the world. In the United States alone, it is reported that over 600,000 Americans succumb to kidney failure.

These stats are alarming, so it is necessary to take proper care of your kidneys, starting with a kidney-friendly diet. These recipes are ideal for whether you have been diagnosed with a kidney problem or want to prevent any kidney issue.

Regarding your well-being and health, it's a smart thought to see your doctor as frequently as conceivable to ensure you don't run into preventable issues that you needn't get. The kidneys are your body's toxin channel (just like the liver), cleaning the blood of remote substances and toxins discharged from things like preservatives in food & other toxins. When you eat flippantly, you fill your body with toxins: either from nourishment, drinks (liquor or alcohol, for instance), or even from the air you inhale (free radicals are in the sun and move through your skin, through dirty air, and numerous food sources contain them). In general, your body will convert innumerable things that appear to be benign until your body's organs convert them into something like formaldehyde because of a synthetic response and transforming phase.

One case of this is a large portion of those diet sugars utilized in diet soft drinks; for instance, Aspartame transforms into formaldehyde in the body. These toxins must be expelled, or they can prompt ailment, renal (kidney) failure, malignant growth, and various other painful problems.

This condition doesn't occur without any forethought; it is an emotional issue, and in that it very well may be both found early and treated, diet changed, and settling what is causing the issue is conceivable. It's conceivable to have partial renal failure, yet, as a rule, it requires some time (or downright awful diet for a short time) to arrive at absolute renal failure. You would prefer not to reach total renal failure since this will require standard dialysis treatments to save your life.

Dialysis treatments explicitly clean the blood of waste and toxins in the blood utilizing a machine because your body can no longer carry out the responsibility. Without treatments, you could die a very painful death. Renal failure can be the consequence of long-haul diabetes, hypertension, unreliable diet, and can stem from other health concerns.

A renal diet is tied in with directing the intake of protein and phosphorus in your eating routine. Restricting your sodium intake is likewise significant. By controlling these two variables, you can control the vast majority of the toxins/waste made by your body. Thus, this enables your kidney to 100% function. If you get this early enough and truly moderate your diets with extraordinary consideration, you could avert all-out renal failure. If you get this early, you can take out the issue completely.

Thank you

Susan Cooper

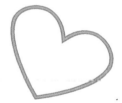

CPSIA information can be obtained
at www.ICGtesting.com
Printed in the USA
BVHW052014300321
603712BV00004B/243

9 781802 351040